Getting Started as a

Pharmacy Preceptor

D0254740

Notice

The author, editor, and publisher have made every effort to ensure the accuracy and completeness of the information presented in this book. However, the author, editor, and publisher cannot be held responsible for the continued currency of the information, any inadvertent errors or omissions, or the application of this information. Therefore, the author, editor, and publisher shall have no liability to any person or entity with regard to claims, loss, or damage caused or alleged to be caused, directly or indirectly, by the use of information contained herein.

Getting Started as a
Pharmacy Preceptor

Randell E. Doty, PharmD

Associate Dean for Experiential Education
College of Pharmacy
University of Florida
Gainesville, Florida

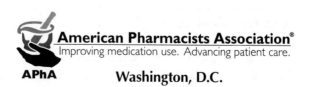

American Pharmacists Association®
Improving medication use. Advancing patient care.

APhA   **Washington, D.C.**

Managing and Content Editor: Vicki Meade, Meade Communications
Acquiring Editor: Sandra Cannon
Proofreader: Cathi Dunn MacRae
Indexer: Jennifer Burton, Columbia Indexing Group
Cover Designer: Scott Neitzke, APhA Creative Services
Layout and Graphics: Michele A. Danoff, Graphics by Design
Case Study Illustrations: Barry Edwards

© 2011 by the American Pharmacists Association
APhA was founded in 1852 as the American Pharmaceutical Association.

Published by the American Pharmacists Association
2215 Constitution Avenue, N.W.
Washington, DC 20037-2985
www.pharmacist.com
www.pharmacylibrary.com

To comment on this book via email, send your message to the publisher at
aphabooks@aphanet.org.

All rights reserved.

*No part of this book may be reproduced, stored in a retrieval system,
or transmitted in any form or by any means, electronic, mechanical,
photocopying, recording, or otherwise, without written permission from the
publisher.*

Library of Congress Cataloging-in-Publication Data

Doty, Randell E.
  Getting started as a pharmacy preceptor / by Randell E. Doty.
    p. ; cm.
  Includes index.
  ISBN 978-1-58212-146-8
  1. Pharmacy--Study and teaching. 2. Preceptorship. I. American Pharma-
cists Association. II. Title.
  [DNLM: 1. Education, Pharmacy. 2. Preceptorship. QV 20]
  RS101.D68 2011
  615'.1076--dc22
                              2010053035

How to Order This Book
Online: www.pharmacist.com/shop_apha
By phone: 800-878-0729 (from the United States and Canada)
VISA®, MasterCard®, and American Express® cards accepted

Dedication

Thanks to my wife Donna for her love and support.

Contents

Case Studies

Preface

For the many readers out there who don't know me, here's a little about myself to help you understand where I'm coming from with this book. I've been the associate dean for experiential education at the University of Florida (UF) College of Pharmacy for 18 years, a position that, as with many things in my life, I came to through serendipity.

I graduated with my PharmD degree from the University of Tennessee (UT) College of Pharmacy in 1988 and then did a residency at the VA Medical Center in Memphis. In my undergrad years I discovered a significant affinity for computers. Throughout pharmacy school I continued this interest and strengthened my skills. When I graduated from UT and went into my residency program, I was already looking for positions where I could combine my interests in pharmacy and computers.

As it happens, toward the end of my residency the director got a call from someone at UF who was looking to fill a faculty position in the Center for Computer Applications in Pharmacy. The people on each end of that phone call knew each other only through a national committee in the VA system. It was a "What the heck? Might as well," call. Serendipity.

I was hired after the interview and started in the summer of 1989. For the next two years, I exercised both skill sets—designing computer interfaces for clinical and educational software—but then, in the post–Gulf War recession, the university came under state budget cuts. Although the center was funded through contracts that covered programmers and other staff, the college of pharmacy could no longer support the faculty positions, and the center was closed.

I needed a new job. The experiential programs director position had just opened up, and it was offered to me. Serendipity.

I decided to take it, but at first wasn't sure if I would stay. Soon I realized how much I enjoyed the teaching aspect of the position. I started reflecting on my relationship to education. My father is a minister and a marriage and family counselor. My mother has been an elementary school teacher and principal. My sister, a former elementary school teacher, now has her PhD in educational development. It was only natural for me to end up in education. Serendipity.

I don't mean to harp on the serendipity issue. Call it fate, design, or an interesting confluence of events. For me it's about grabbing opportunities when they come by. Writing this book is another example.

Over my 18 years in experiential education I have seen our college go from a BS/PharmD curriculum with 90 students per class, 60% of whom were BS students, to an entry-level PharmD program with 300 students per class. During this time, amazing people have helped me learn to do what I do. These include Ron Stewart, Tom Munyer, David Angaran, Pete Pevonka, Jeff Delafuente, Diane Beck, Dan Robinson, Mike McKenzie, Bill Riffee, and many others. The end result of all they've taught me is who I am today. Now you know who to blame.

I tried to write this book like a conversation—as if you and I are sitting down somewhere talking about what you need to do to be a preceptor. It's a conversation I've had many times, made up of pieces of knowledge pulled from all those people mentioned above as well as input from others over the years. Although you're not able to talk with all the people who've mentored me, you can pick up bits of their advice in the pages of this book.

What does all this mean for you? It means that this book is different from other books and articles on precepting. Instead of covering everything you'd ever want to know about clinical teaching and precepting from an academic point of view, it's more of a "This Old House" for precepting. If you are really busy, need to get started fast, want quick answers, or seek a bit of advice, this is the book for you.

Randell Doty
December 2010

Introduction

Getting Started as a Pharmacy Preceptor explores the What, When, How, and Why of precepting students. The chapters are arranged chronologically to take you from the point where you decide to precept to the point where you are deeply involved in educating students.

The book's primary focus is advanced pharmacy practice experiences (APPEs), but its advice and information should be applicable to introductory pharmacy practice experiences (IPPEs) as well. The latter part of the book looks at student problems in two ways. Chapter 9 points out overarching principles useful when dealing with student issues. It leads into eight case studies covering a variety of problems that can occur with students in practical training.

What Is a Preceptor?

It would be a good idea to get on the same page about what a preceptor is. The term gets used regularly but is rarely defined in a meaningful way. In short, a preceptor is a teacher, instructor, and coach who moves students from knowledge to application to integration in a practical training environment. Preceptors help students go from the "head knowledge" they get in the classroom to being able to apply that knowledge in practice and take care of real patients.

In IPPEs, preceptors focus mostly on direct instruction and helping students apply knowledge to simple patient care situations. In APPEs, preceptors help students integrate their knowledge and apply it to caring for complex patients.

The precepting concept is not new. Helping people make the transition from knowledgeable but unskilled to knowledgeable and skilled has been part of the teacher–student paradigm throughout history. Wherever failing a task involves serious consequences, someone has stepped in to say, "Let me show you. Then see how you do before you try it on your own."

I tell my students the following story to introduce them to why the precepting relationship is important.

> You have to fly across the country. On the day of your flight you arrive at the airport and go through all the customary checks. As you stand in line to take your seat, you pause near the front of the plane, where you can see into the cockpit, and you hear the pilots talking. You listen to a bit of the preflight check and hear the following conversation:

> **Pilot:** "Wow. I am really excited about today's flight!"
> **Copilot:** "Really, why?"
> **Pilot:** "Well, this is my first actual flight in a real airplane. I have done many hours in simulations but never in a real plane before."
> **Copilot:** "That *is* exciting!"
> **Pilot:** "Yes, the simulations are great, but I am guessing that actually taking off and landing are going to be amazing!"

> At this point, you can either go to your seat or run screaming from the plane. Which would you choose?

By telling this story, I remind students where they are in their training. They are still untested. Until they have been under the watchful eye of an actual practitioner who can see them perform and sign off on their ability to do so, they are just like that pilot and have no business flying that plane. The knowledge and expertise of a seasoned pilot will turn the untrained into the trained and deliver to the public someone they can trust with their lives. This is what it means to be a preceptor.

What You Must Do: The Gist

When you become a preceptor, you'll work with three parties to accomplish your objectives: your student, your practice site's health care team, and the college or colleges of pharmacy placing students with you. The three primary things you'll need to do well when working with these parties are to communicate, communicate, communicate.

For the student you must:

- Communicate objectives.
- Provide a thorough orientation.

- Give regular feedback.
- Provide a thorough and accurate evaluation.

For the school you must:

- Obtain the required documents.
- Stay on top of the schedule of students.
- Watch for deadlines.
- Keep in touch when problems occur.

For the health care team you must:

- Set expectations for their participation.
- Create an environment for the free flow of information.
- Set limits for the team and student.

The chapters and case studies that follow explore topics related to the points above and provide tips and lessons that two decades of overseeing experiential education programs have taught me.

Chapter 1

Are You Precepting for the Right Reasons?

In my experience, the single biggest indicator of successful precepting is your personal desire to do it well. If you are choosing to precept students for the right reasons, most likely you will become an excellent preceptor. If not, you will find yourself on the wrong end of the student rumor mill soon enough. So...

What are the right reasons?

- Because you want to influence future pharmacists.
- Because you have skills that you believe you could teach well to others.
- Because you have an internal desire to help other pharmacists learn how to take care of patients in your specialty area.
- Because you want to give back to the profession.
- Because you remember the value you got from your preceptors and want to provide the same value to today's students.
- Because you feel that bringing students into your practice site will extend your reach and increase the ability to provide quality patient care.

And what are the wrong reasons?

- Because your manager wants you to.
- Because the person who was in your position before you was a preceptor.
- Because you like the benefits from the school.
- Because it looks good on your curriculum vitae or résumé.
- Because you could use some help when it gets busy.
- Because you are loyal to your alma mater.

The Good, the Bad, and the Reality

A nice thing about the good reasons is that they trump the poor ones. That is, if you're motivated to be a preceptor by the reasons in the first list, it doesn't matter if some reasons in the second list apply to you, too.

If the only reasons you want to be a preceptor are in the second list, you might as well stop reading now. Maybe you can give this book to someone else. But before you do, think about whether you know *for certain* what your reasons are.

> The single biggest indicator of successful precepting is your personal desire to do it well.

I have found that sometimes people choose to become preceptors for the wrong reasons only to find out later that they have a passion for it. So maybe your key reason right now is that you have been asked to be a preceptor by a supervisor, or some experiential director at the school where you're an alumnus smooth-talked you into it. Even so, it may be the stimulus you need to find out that "right reasons" are true as well.

Do You Have Doubts?

If you're uncertain whether being a preceptor is right for you, think about this. Is it possible that, not having been exposed to the process of providing clinical education as a preceptor, you're unaware that a clinical teacher is lurking inside you? It warrants a trial to find out if that lurker will emerge. Among the entire population of preceptors, most likely had no idea before they got started how much they'd like it and the positive effects they'd have on others. You could turn out to be a star.

It seems to me that the risk–reward equation is stacked pretty well in favor of trying out the preceptor role. In the worst case, you find out after a few students that precepting is not for you, and you stop. A few students will have had a mediocre experience—not great, but not devastating.

In the best case, you find out that you really enjoy it and are good at it. If that happens, literally hundreds of future pharmacists will benefit from your guidance. That sounds like a positive balance to me.

Broadening Your Impact on Patients

One last note regarding why to be a preceptor: From a patient care perspective, an individual practitioner can help only a limited number of patients in a single day, month, or year. As a preceptor, every student you train becomes an extension of your ability to care for patients. A multiplier, if you will. After several years your students will also have students, and the effect is further multiplied.

If you are truly invested in improving the outcomes of patients, there is no better use of your time than training other practitioners to do just that.

Now that I've been a preceptor for many years, I occasionally get to trace a practitioner-training lineage back to its source, and it is a thing of beauty. The line of quality that extends forward from preceptor to student, and backward from that same preceptor to his or her teachers, is easier to identify in residency programs, but it exists with preceptors in introductory and advanced pharmacy practice experiences (IPPEs and APPEs) as well. It is the genealogy of our profession.

> As a preceptor, every student you train becomes an extension of your ability to care for patients.

For example, two of my colleagues, Paul Doering and Randy Hatton, codirected the drug information service at Shands Hospital for many years. As I write this, Paul is getting ready to retire, but Randy is still precepting pharmacy students. Over the past 20 years they have precepted roughly 480 students and 20 residents. One of their students and residents, Bernadette Belgado, is now director of the drug information service for Shands Jacksonville. Over the last 10 years she has precepted about 250 students. She is just one of their former students, and certainly not everyone who comes through their program goes on to teach clinically—or to match their pace, if they do—but even if just two or three a year become preceptors, the number of people Paul and Randy will have influenced is amazing. Your potential for affecting our profession is no different.

Take a moment and think about your own training. Who influenced the way you practice? And who influenced those people? You can picture the genealogy stretching behind you, fanning out like a tree. Becoming a preceptor is your step toward having it reach forward—and forming healthy new branches.

Chapter 2

What Can You Do?

Basically, pharmacy schools offer two kinds of experiential education.

- Introductory pharmacy practice experiences (IPPEs) take place while students are in the earlier years of their pharmacy education.
- Advanced pharmacy practice experiences (APPEs) typically occur in the final year of pharmacy school.

Depending on your setting, your responsibilities, and the kind of time you have available, you may precept one or the other, or even both.

What Fits You Best?

Here are some things to consider to determine which of the two types of practice experiences might fit you best as a preceptor.

Considerations Regarding IPPEs

- Students have less experience and tend to require more supervision for difficult tasks.
- The competencies students are developing are typically for the baseline of practice rather than for specialty areas.
- Depending on the university requirements, students' time with you may be intermittent over a semester or blocked into a few weeks.
- Time on site is often fairly rigid, for a specific number of hours at predetermined times.
- Because each student's experience before pharmacy school varies widely, those taking part in an IPPE may have a wide range of baseline knowledge and abilities.
- Usually, an IPPE requires time in both a community setting and a hospital setting, although other options may be available depending on how the curriculum is designed at each pharmacy school.

Considerations Regarding APPEs

- Students are meant to experience the breadth and depth of possible skills in a given practice arena.
- Competencies for students in APPEs are designed to prepare them for entry-level practice. Thus the site and patient base must allow students to expand their knowledge and skills.
- Students' time at the site is typically four to eight weeks.
- Students are not limited to an eight-hour day. I tell my students that APPEs *start out* at 40 hours per week and *go up* from there.
- APPE sites need to reinforce general patient care principles with rigor, or they must provide an opportunity to explore in detail a specialized practice environment or specialized patient base.
- APPEs can occur almost anywhere pharmacy is practiced.

What's in a Name?

A brief note on nomenclature. Over the years, the experiential portion of pharmacy training has been referred to as many things: an internship, externship, clerkship, practicum, rotation, etc. In recent years the Accreditation Council for Pharmacy Education has emphasized using the standard language listed above: IPPE and APPE.

The problem is, it's hard to undo years of habit. So, if you're around any preceptors or faculty who've been around for a while (old guys and gals), you may hear other terms being tossed around interchangeably. Just smile, nod, and ask for clarification if you are unsure what they are talking about.

Identifying Learning Opportunities

One thing I find when talking to preceptors is that they often underestimate the opportunities at their site for student learning. I'm not sure if this is because they're unclear about what the curriculum requires or because they have biases about the activities that are appropriate for students to participate in.

I suggest that you take time to brainstorm about the possibilities before deciding where and how students will be included. If you work with a team, you should involve them in this exercise. If you practice alone, brainstorming is a bit harder, but you can contact folks in similar practice areas to find out what they do with the students they precept.

The underlying purpose of the exercise should be to create a list of all the possible functions in your practice site. Maybe even include some in which you are not currently able to participate. Having a student may open them up. Once you have this long list of opportunities, you can work on narrowing it down.

Don't Overlook Valuable Learning

Be careful about the narrowing, though. Some preceptors seem to want to isolate students from certain tasks. I will give you an example.

> Preceptors often under-estimate the opportunities at their site for student learning.

One preceptor told me that he allocated time in the afternoon for students to work in the library on projects because there was nothing going on for them otherwise at the practice site. The idea of setting aside time to focus on projects is not bad, per se, but knowing what I know, I wanted to see if this student might be missing out on something valuable.

So I asked what the preceptor was doing during that time. He said that this is when he works on reports and committee assignments. I asked if knowing how to work on those reports and understanding how those committees function was not worth learning. As it turns out, those things *were* worth learning, but in the preceptor's mind, they were not "fun" activities, so he isolated the student from them.

This kind of thinking can leave out very valuable opportunities to build skills and be exposed to important tasks. Remember, we are training people to be pharmacists. Pharmacists carry out both patient care and non-patient care duties.

If you're still having trouble determining which activities are appropriate for your students, talk to someone at the college of pharmacy. Describe what you do and what a student could be involved with. The college will help you decide.

On a general note, if you ever get stuck, call the college. That's what it's there for.

Calculating Numbers

The question of how many students your site can accommodate comes up quite a bit in decisions about providing clinical education. Do you have the space, time, and patient load to accommodate one student at a time, two, or several? Important considerations are covered below.

What Does the Law Allow?

Every state's laws are different. You will need to explore how many students are allowed at your site based on where you are practicing. The experiential director at the university should be able to help answer this question, but be ready for some ambiguity.

State laws and regulations regarding the practice of pharmacy and the presence of pharmacy students in the practice setting often have holes in their coverage. Some laws apply only to dispensing areas. What does that mean when the rotation the student is involved in does not have a dispensing area? Some laws refer only to the absolute ratio of pharmacists to nonpharmacists, whether that nonpharmacist is a technician, clerk, or student, not to a ratio of pharmacist to specific type of supervisee. Some laws clearly differentiate between students, techs, and clerks in regard to supervision.

If the experiential director can't help you, ask others who have similar programs what they do. If that doesn't work, ask the board of pharmacy—but keep in mind that boards of pharmacy are government bureaucracies. When faced with a gray area that is hard to research, they may simply err on the side of caution and say "no" to your question.

What Does the Space Allow?

Every site is different. You will need to assess just how many physical bodies can occupy the environment.

- How many workstations are available?
- How many chairs?
- Where will the students be spending most of their time?

Having a small office does not matter if you are never there. If most of the work takes place away from the office, you can have quite a bit of flexibility. In today's world, instead of thinking about *where* the work gets done, we can focus on the fact that it *gets* done.

What Does the Workload Allow?

In considering this question, the time of year makes a difference. Some experiences may have a seasonal nature. For example, cities in the heart of Florida double or triple their populations during the winter, changing the hospital census and the need for students at the site. In other locations, the hospital census is consistent year-round. In either case, the workload is an indicator of the number of opportunities available for students. You may not be able to tell for sure what the workload allows until you have had a few students.

How Effectively Can You Teach More Than One Student?

This question is hard for anyone to answer other than you, and it may take some trial and error. I find that preceptors generally choose to work with only one student because they are unsure of the time commitment. I like to point out that economy of scale factors into clinical training. If you are going to have a topic discussion with one student, you can just as easily have it with two or even three.

Likewise, if you have only one student and she has a question, she has only one source for the answer. You. If you have two students, they will ask each other the question first and come to you only when they both don't know the answer.

> Do you have the space, time, and patient load to accommodate one student at a time, two, or several?

Having said that, I know that not everyone can handle multiple students. If the issues above regarding law, space, and workload prevent bringing on more than one student at a time, it matters very little if you'd prefer to precept several.

When Is the Right Time?

You must think about the variations in your site from month to month. Does every month offer the same opportunities for student learning experiences? If your site is fairly consistent, you may be able to accommodate a student every month—and, in fact, you may prefer a constant student presence because it allows you to get more done. If so, contact the college to determine the feasibility.

The type of experience you offer, whether this type of experience is in demand among students, and your location all play a role in whether the college can provide you with a full schedule of students. For example, if the experience you provide is required for all students and is located in a highly populated area, and if a limited number of sites also provide this type of experience, accommodating your request will be much more likely. If, however, you offer an elective experience in a small rural community far from a population center or in an area where multiple sites provide a similar experience, the likelihood of obtaining a full schedule of students is probably low.

If patient load or activity level varies at your site based on the time of year, you will need to decide which months you want to have students and which months will not work. Other things to consider:

- Staffing levels
- Vacations
- Scheduled state, regional, or national meetings
- Other significant events

You may also want to build in some "time out" from having students, particularly if you are precepting on your own and not as part of a team. When precepting solo, taking on too many students can lead to some degree of burnout—a problem you can prevent by planning breaks.

The Scheduling Process

No matter what kind of learning experience you eventually decide to offer, you need a process in place to match the students to the site. At most pharmacy schools, this process is typically handled by the director of experiential education, who is faced with the daunting task of ensuring that students get the kinds of experiential training they need to fulfill their requirements, based on the experience types available. Although it's not necessary for you to grasp all the nuances of how this process works, a few important things to understand are discussed below.

Opt In or Opt Out

Each college has a mechanism to collect data from you about your availability. If you don't tell the college if you are available or not, the experiential director can't know whether to schedule students with you. Some colleges may work on an *opt-in* method and some on an *opt-out* method. (I'm not sure anyone uses these exact terms, but for the sake of discussion, we'll use them here.)

Colleges that operate on an opt-in methodology will want you to let them know each cycle if you are available, how many opportunities you are willing to offer, when, and how many students for each. Colleges that operate on an *opt-out* method will assume you are in for a standard setup—such as whatever you offered the previous year, or whatever standard package of numbers and dates the college uses when a rotation site does not specify what it wants, such as "one student a month for every month."

It is important that you know which method you are dealing with. If you think it is *opt-in* and it is actually *opt-out*, you may end up with students assigned to you that you were not expecting. If you think it is *opt-out* when it is actually *opt-in*, you could find yourself with no students at all.

As a first-time preceptor, it's best not to assume anything. Get in touch with the college and ask, for example, "What would be the best way for me to let you know when I would like to have students, and how many, for the next APPE cycle?" Then be specific about what you're offering, to help ensure you get exactly what you want.

> The type of experience you offer, whether this type of experience is in demand among students, and your location all play a role in whether the college can provide you with a full schedule of students.

Experiential Directors Are Not Perfect

Far from it, in fact. And although most experiential directors use some kind of computer system to make the scheduling process easier, none of these systems is perfect, either. For the system to operate correctly, the data entered into it must be accurate and the user must avoid making mistakes.

Eventually something will go wrong, and when it does, it's helpful if you can be patient while corrections are made. Also, once the schedule is made available, it's very important that you check it closely for errors. Make sure it matches up with your expectations. The people doing the scheduling have so much information to work with, they are unable to pick out every error. So please point out when they mess up.

For example, I have 300 students who must do APPEs each year over the course of 11 months, and these students all have very specific ideas of where they want to be and when. And I have approximately 1600 active preceptors with very specific ideas of when they want students and how many; some have additional prerequisites to comply with. Overall, that adds up to 3300 experiences and countless requirements to be met. Some of them are not going to be right and when that happens, the college needs to hear from you as soon as possible.

Your Rotation Is Part of the Whole

A student's experiential education is made up of many parts beyond the specific experience you offer. A balanced "whole" composed of different experiences is what's most important. Requirements set by the Accreditation Council for Pharmacy Education (ACPE) and individual colleges attempt to ensure that this balance occurs.

Each APPE provides knowledge, skills, and attitudes (KSAs) that will be valuable to students in their career. For APPE schedules, I look at the overall balance of a schedule rather than at individual rotations to see what the student is getting. Sometimes this is a hard concept to get across to students. I use the concept of personality testing, which most people are familiar with, to help explain. By looking at rotations as if they have a personality, I can define them using the following attributes.

- **General knowledge, skills, and attitudes.** These are the underpinnings of practice. Education items fall in this category if they are useful in virtually any setting and can also be gained in most settings.

- **Unique knowledge, skills, and attitudes.** These education items provide breadth of experience. They are found only in certain practice settings or among certain patient types and are typically only useful in specific areas, but can translate to other unique areas.

- **Patient interaction.** This category involves actual patient interaction and caregiving. Standing at a bedside while the patient is nonresponsive counts as this type of activity, but communicating with patients in a meaningful way counts much more. Likewise, phone conversations count, but person-to-person conversations count more because they include nonverbal communication.

- **Problem frequency.** This category refers to the rate at which problems occur at the site. It has to do with repetition and the degree to which students can become comfortable and confident in their use of certain skills. I like to think of this category and the next one as involving brain-building exercises—reinforcing knowledge and skills so they are ready for action when needed. Another good analogy is exercising a muscle. Repetition builds definition.

- **Problem complexity.** This category refers to the difficulty of problems that occur at the site. How hard is each problem to solve? How many resources does each one take to solve? How many possible viable solutions are there? How hard will it be to implement? Complexity builds new abilities and creates new pathways for problem solving so students have alternate methods to draw from when their first approach does not work.

- **Autonomy.** This category involves the amount of responsibility students are given. Within the limits of supervision, how accountable are students for outcomes? Autonomy is necessary for students to eventually transition to being independent practitioners.

Each rotation will involve different amounts of these attributes. A community experience, for example, will probably have a great deal of general KSAs, some unique KSAs, a good amount of patient interaction and problem frequency, a smaller amount of problem complexity, and some autonomy. A critical-care rotation, on the other hand, will have some general KSAs, quite a bit of unique KSAs, a very small amount of patient interaction, high problem frequency and complexity, and low autonomy.

You can probably estimate the mix and volume of attributes for your own rotation and for others you're familiar with—which constitutes the rotation's "personality." A schedule has a personality, too, which is the aggregate of all rotations included in it. The student benefits from all the rotations to achieve his or her education outcome.

The point of this discussion is to emphasize that no rotation provides everything. If a schedule is not balanced to cover everything a student needs to learn, it's not your obligation to make up the slack. And you may not be equipped to. Furthermore, if you try to make up the slack, your student may miss out on the very thing your site is good at providing.

Of course, if you see a deficit in a student's experience and have the means to help, you should, but remember that you are not alone—practice sites in other rotations may be better equipped to help the student.

Don't be surprised if the "balance" concept is not articulated by everyone in terms of personality attributes. This is my way of explaining things. I hope it has been helpful.

Chapter 3

Getting Ready

Now that you've decided to become a preceptor, it's time to contact your local pharmacy school or college to let them know you're available and to discover the next steps. Your best starting point is the office that handles experiential programs, which may go by different names depending on the school. Typically the title of the person in charge of these programs is "director of experiential programs" or "director of experiential education." The school's website should have a link that connects to experiential education information and a way to send an inquiry by email.

Questions to Ask the College

Important questions you should ask when you contact the college for more information about precepting include:

- How do I become a preceptor for your school? Ask about either introductory pharmacy practice experiences (IPPEs) or advanced pharmacy practice experiences (APPEs), depending on your choice.
- What paperwork do I need to complete?
- Do you have a manual for clinical faculty?
- Do you have sample syllabi for the kind of experience I will offer?
- Do you have preceptor training I can complete?
- How do I let you know of my availability?
- What are the timelines for completing the necessary steps?

Setting the Stage

In getting ready for your first student, the tasks involved depend on what the college provides. Even if your first student won't join you for a year, it's best to go ahead and start planning the rotation. Among items you should make sure are in place before your first student arrives on site:

- An affiliation agreement between your practice site and the college.
- A syllabus outlining the objectives, activities, and evaluation criteria for the experience.
- Introductory correspondence to provide to students containing the information they need to get started.
- An orientation plan for the first day.
- A calendar with key dates and activities in the rotation.
- Forms or assessment tools you will use.

Affiliation Agreements

Colleges and corporations sometimes call these agreements by different names, but basically they are a contract between the two parties outlining the responsibilities of each and what happens if things go wrong, such as the circumstances under which a student can be dismissed and the site's responsibility if a student is injured on the job. If the college and the preceptor's employer agree to use one or the other's standard agreement, it simplifies the process. If someone wants changes, be prepared for a wait. The attorneys for both groups will get involved, and the process can really drag on.

> Make sure you are aware of the human resources requirements for students at your site.

Try to avoid being the middleman between your legal department and the one at the college. Sometimes it's inevitable that you will be forced into that role, but most of the time, if you can convince the lawyers to talk to each other, everything moves along faster.

Make sure you are aware of the human resources (HR) requirements for students at your site. Because the Joint Commission (formerly the Joint Commission on Accreditation of Healthcare Organizations) requires students at the site to meet the same standards as employees, HR requirements are usually included in the affiliation agreement if it comes from your company, but they are not included if the agreement comes from the college.

Having clear requirements helps minimize confusion. Among questions the HR requirements should address:

- Are drug screens required?
- Tuberculosis skin tests?

- Background checks?
- If any of the above are required, what will you and the student need to do to coordinate them?

The pharmacy college will have dealt with these matters at many sites already. If you are part of a larger organization, most likely the processes you need are in place. If you are not, ask the college about the processes it uses for other organizations. There is really no need to start from scratch if something is already established that works well.

Syllabus

Your syllabus is the roadmap for your rotation. If your roadmap is not detailed enough, students will lose their way, so spend time up front making sure it covers everything you need. On a very basic level a syllabus is important for three reasons:

1. To provide clarity regarding the purpose of the learning experience.
2. To provide structure.
3. To make the evaluation criteria clear and specific.

Before creating your syllabus, ask your pharmacy college if they have a template, or gather from colleagues samples you can use as a model. Figure 3-1 provides a rough template for an APPE syllabus. Now, let's look at constructing your syllabus point by point.

The Header

Your syllabus should display prominently at the top the key identifiers that let readers know immediately which IPPE or APPE it relates to. Because this document will be one of many delivered to the college, as well as to students individually, it must be easily identified. Make sure you include:

- The rotation name, including the name of the site and type of experience.
- The name of the preceptor(s) and other contact people for the experience.
- Goals/description for the experience. Treat this like an abstract for the experience, with a paragraph or two describing basic things the student will learn and do. This description comes in handy if the college also needs a short overview for a website or catalog that details opportunities for students researching experiential learning options.

Figure 3-1 | Syllabus Template for an APPE

Below is a simple template for an APPE syllabus, which provides a good starting point if you don't have other examples. Notes and instructions are in italics.

Advanced Pharmacy Practice Experience Syllabus   HEADER
for
Rotation Name
Preceptor Name(s)

Goals of the Experience:

Include a short overview of what the experience entails and what the student should learn by participating. It would start out something like this:

> The goal of this APPE is to expose the student to patient care in a *[fill in blank]* setting. Through their participation, students will gain the knowledge, skills, and attitudes necessary to… *[fill in to capture the big picture of the experience].*

Outcomes/Objectives: BODY

List a number of outcomes for the experience. Most colleges prefer an ability-based outcome (ABO) format, which is composed of knowledge, skills, and attitudes. Below, the ABO is in bold and individual objectives follow in a list. You probably need only three to five ABOs for most APPEs. If you struggle with the ABOs, try writing individual objectives first and then group them logically to identify common themes.

- **Students should be able to identify and utilize drug information services to facilitate their role as a drug information specialist for other health care professionals and patients to achieve positive therapeutic outcomes.**
  - ➤ Interact appropriately with other members of the health care team.
  - ➤ Know and use sources of drug information for any given patient care area.
  - ➤ Apply drug information to obtain positive outcomes for patients.
  - ➤ Serve as drug information specialists for patients and other health care professionals.

- **Students should be able to develop oral or written presentations on drug-related topics for other health care professionals and patients.**
  - ➤ Effectively communicate in verbal and/or written form, in concise and organized fashion, a pharmaceutical evaluation of the patient.

Figure 3-1 | *continued*

> Serve as drug information specialists for patients and other health care professionals.
> Develop presentation skills for various audiences for interdisciplinary education.
> Develop communication skills for patient education.

Activities/Projects:

List activities the student will perform. Although you can organize the list however you wish, sorting activities into daily, weekly, one-time, intermittent, and optional categories will make it easier for you to create your calendar later. This list can be quite long. Create something like the following list, but with specific details instead of generalities:

- Activity 1, Daily *[maybe a patient care activity]*
- Activity 2, Daily *[maybe a quality assurance activity]*
- Activity 3, Weekly *[maybe a journal club]*
- Activity 4, Twice Weekly *[maybe a disease topic presentation]*
- Activity 5, One Time *[maybe a formal oral presentation to staff]*

Evaluation Criteria:

Include the evaluation techniques that will be used and when. Also include the overall course evaluation's grading criteria, weighting, and grading scale. The last two are commonly dictated by the college, but if they aren't, include your own.

- Daily Activity 1 & 2 will be evaluated by direct observation from the preceptor, as well as reports of performance from other health care team members collected periodically throughout the rotation.
- Weekly Activity 1 & 2 will be evaluated by all present at the event using the following specific criteria… *[include the criteria]*.
- One-Time Activity 1 will be evaluated by all preceptors and residents attending the presentation using the following criteria…*[include the criteria. If a separate form is needed, place it at the end as an appendix]*.

Figure 3-1 | *continued*

- A formal midpoint evaluation will be conducted using the following weighting:

  ➢ Activity 1   35%
  ➢ Activity 2   15%
  ➢ Activity 3   10%
  ➢ Activity 4   10%
  ➢ Activity 5   10%
  ➢ Professionalism   20%

It is okay to include overall issues that are not specific to a particular activity but common to all.

- Grading Scale

  ➢ A >90
  ➢ B >80
  ➢ C >70
  ➢ D >60
  ➢ F <60

This grading scale is simple, but not all are. Some colleges use a pass/fail system.

Attendance: FOOTER

Insert canned attendance policy from the college here.

Student Conduct Guidelines:

These could include many things. Here are some examples:

- The student must exhibit a professional appearance in manner and dress.
- The student must adhere to the standards of dress and behavior specified by the instructor to whom he or she is assigned. These standards should be identical to those required of all pharmacists in the pharmacy.
- The student shall identify himself or herself as a student at all times.
- Academic honesty is expected. Any lapses in academic honesty will be subject to the processes dictated by the student's university.

Figure 3-1 | *continued*

- The student is obligated to respect any and all confidences revealed during the assignment in pharmacy records, medical records, fee systems, professional policies, etc.
- The student must keep in mind that the primary objective of APPEs is learning and that learning is not a passive process but requires a deep and active commitment on the student's part.
- The student should recognize that the optimum learning experience requires mutual respect and courtesy between the instructor and himself or herself.
- The student should encourage communication with all persons involved in the APPE including the instructor, physicians, other health professionals, and patients.
- When making professional judgments the student should first discuss alternatives with the instructor.
- The student is responsible for adhering to the work schedule of the instructor. For the student's own benefit, it may be necessary at times to devote more than the scheduled time or to deviate from the schedule.
- The student should be punctual in meeting the schedule and is obligated to notify the instructor as soon as possible if he or she will be absent or late.

<u>Student Evaluations of APPE and Preceptor:</u>

Colleges may have a specific statement they want you to use here. If not, here is something that will probably work. Adjust as needed.

Students will comply with the guidelines from their home university for submitting faculty and APPE evaluations. Because evaluations are the cornerstone for improving the experience, the faculty for this APPE are very interested in hearing your opinion. Please feel free to provide feedback throughout the experience, as well. It may not be possible to make changes midstream, but we would still like your input.

<u>Background Material:</u>

List training materials, journal articles, guidelines, book chapters, etc. that you want students to read or complete prior to beginning your experience.

- Reading 1
- Reading 2

Figure 3-1 | *continued*

Additional Requirements:

List tools and equipment students need to be successful, such as laptop, handheld device, calculator, etc.

- Requirement 1
- Requirement 2

Access to Site Benefits:

List site-specific benefits that students have access to and procedures they need to follow, such as:

- While on this APPE, students have access to the following:
  - ➢ Free parking in the employee garage. The HR department will issue you a pass on the first day.
  - ➢ One free meal in the cafeteria each day. Other meals are at normal prices. Swipe your hospital ID to access this benefit. Your ID will be made for you on the first day.

Accommodations:

Many times, specific language is necessary here regarding the Americans with Disabilities Act. Check with the university.

Frequently Asked Questions:

This section can be added to, as needed.

The Body

The core of your syllabus should contain three types of information:

1. Objectives (what you want students to learn).
2. Activities (what they are going to do).
3. Evaluation Criteria (how you are going to document their learning).

A very effective way to construct this part of your syllabus and make sure it is complete is to link these three items so you are sure every objective has an activity, every activity has a way to be evaluated, etc.

Try actually drawing a line from one to the other, as in a matching question on a test, to connect objectives, activities, and evaluation criteria. If an item doesn't have lines going or coming to corresponding pieces, you need to investigate the problem and ask yourself whether that item should be part of your syllabus.

> When constructing objectives, try to use words that describe the student's learning in ways that are measurable.

Some Tips on Objectives

As noted at the start of this chapter, you should check with the college to see if they have sample syllabi. If they do, these samples can be a good starting point for constructing yours. The college may even have a syllabus that's required for your specific type of experience.

The format for objectives preferred by many colleges is called an ability-based outcome (ABO). ABOs are explicit statements describing the knowledge, skills, and attitudes students should gain—that is, the outcomes they should achieve—as a result of the learning experience. For someone not paid or trained as an educator, constructing ABOs can be daunting. If the college requires ABOs for your syllabus, put together objectives as best you can and then ask the college for help in organizing them into ABOs.

When constructing your objectives, try to use words that describe the student's learning in ways that are measurable, which is very useful when thinking about how the student will be evaluated on each objective. It's common for people who are inexperienced at writing objectives to use the word "understand," as in: "Upon completion of this experience, the student should be able to understand…" But how do you evaluate whether someone understands? It is difficult. Using words that represent identifiable actions, such as "describe" or "demonstrate," allows you to easily transfer objectives to evaluation techniques. Again, if you get stuck, ask for assistance. Faculty at the college will be happy to help.

Some Tips on Activities

Regarding the activities you will include in your training experience, try to be as comprehensive as possible. Following is a list of the types of activities to consider:

- Patient care activities
- Discussions
- Meetings
- Projects
- Exams
- Papers
- Presentations

Some Tips on Evaluation

Of the two primary types of evaluation, one involves assessing a specific activity or "educational event," such as grading a student's formal oral presentation. The other is a comprehensive evaluation that gives the student an overall grade for the experience. It's best to administer comprehensive evaluations at the midpoint of the experience, and using the same criteria, at the end.

Colleges rarely dictate how you should evaluate specific activities, but some stipulate how you must conduct comprehensive evaluations. At one extreme, the college may require you to follow a very rigid approach; at the other extreme, the college may leave the approach up to you.

Two key trends today are for colleges to:

- Provide preceptors with a template for comprehensive evaluations, which contains specific criteria and tools.
- Cooperate regionally to create a common evaluation system, which simplifies processes for the many preceptors who work with students from multiple pharmacy schools.

These trends have pluses and minuses. On the plus side, you only need to learn and use one system and you don't have to create it yourself. On the minus side, you have to adapt your learning experiences to fit a system designed to be universal, not specific, which can feel awkward. It is a trade-off. On the whole, I think that the plus side wins, but I have to admit some bias in this regard since I participate with a group of colleges that have worked together to create one evaluation system for our region.

If you are working in a cooperative system, get a copy of the evaluation form when you are creating your syllabus, which will help with your objectives and evaluation criteria.

Weighting

Whether you are using a template evaluation system from the college or designing your own, you need to decide, based on the objectives, what you will evaluate and how significant each part is—which is often referred to as "weighting." Weighting a rotation really comes down to defining which parts of the experience are most important. The weight of each item should be clearly spelled out on your syllabus.

Unfortunately, it can be hard to figure out the most important parts. A good exercise to help you determine weighting is to start with checkmarks. Put all your objectives and activities on a page. On another page, list the criteria you will use to identify which activities are most important. Then, on the first page, draw checkmarks next to each item based on your criteria.

For example, apply checkmarks according to how much time is going to be spent in each activity. More checkmarks equals more time. Apply checkmarks to indicate how important each item is to patient care. Add checkmarks for how many times the educational activity might occur, etc. You can even place checkmarks based on how much weight your supervisor attributes to each item in your own evaluations, such as 70% for patient care, 20% for administrative duties, and 10% for personnel supervision.

When you're done, simply looking at the page should give you a good idea of the weights. You can also add up the number of checkmarks next to each category and divide by the total number of checkmarks on the page to get percentages. Of course this exercise might lead to further adjustment, but it's a good way to get started.

Before I make weighting seem too easy, I must mention an issue that can make it more complex: how professional (or unprofessional) behavior is measured.

1. Some colleges build in positive approach—allocating points for attendance, punctuality, professional attire, teamwork, professionalism, enthusiasm, follow-through, etc. If students do well, they earn those points; if they do poorly, they earn few or none.

2. Some colleges deduct points from the final grade if the student fails to meet a baseline level. In other words, you make subtractions at the end of the experience when students fall short in the behaviors and attitudes noted above, such as letter-grade reductions for unexcused absences.

Both of these systems work, but you must know which one the college uses because it will make a big difference in how the rotation is weighted. If the behaviors and attitudes are included in the evaluation, be careful to apply enough weight to them. Otherwise, when a student does poorly on them, he or she will not receive the appropriate points for performance. If you are not sure which way this works for the colleges you're affiliated with, ask.

Evaluating Specific Aspects
In your syllabus, in addition to conveying the weighting and how it relates to the final grade, you should explain how each educational event will be evaluated, such as:

- Direct observation of performance.
- Report of performance to faculty member by other health care team members.
- Formal evaluation of educational presentation.
- Formal oral and/or written testing.

Although some of these approaches may be self-evident, stating them in the syllabus helps the student clearly understand the sources of information that will contribute to the final grade.

Assessing student performance on each educational event calls for tools that can be applied systematically so you get useful, consistent information. Consistent tools are especially important when assessments are conducted by many people, such as other preceptors, residents, and students. You need to be sure that their input is useful and can be easily aggregated.

You can certainly determine the criteria to include and develop your own evaluation tools, but more than likely someone else has created such tools and used them for years with success. Check in with the college, which can either give you examples of tried-and-true tools or supply contact information of preceptors who provide learning experiences similar to yours. Don't be afraid to ask; the college and other preceptors probably collected samples from someone else, too.

The Footer

This section of the syllabus provides policies and "housekeeping" details. For example:

- Attendance policies, including tardiness, authorized absences, holidays, etc. Here you can elaborate on points in the evaluation section, such as emphasizing how attendance affects the final grade.
- Student conduct, including specific policies associated with student attire, confidentiality, adherence to site policies, academic dishonesty, etc. You can elaborate on points in the evaluation section, such as, "Students are expected to perform all activities in concordance with the academic honesty policies of the university. Academic dishonesty will be dealt with as laid out in those policies."
- Procedures for evaluating the instructor and the experience. Each college will have its own policies and will likely supply the evaluation forms and instructions.
- A listing of readings, training programs, videos, or other activities students must complete before the rotation. The list should supply source information for the materials such as websites, books, journals, software, or learning systems.
- A listing of tools that students must have available, such as computers, calculators, hand-held devices, and reference books.
- Information about site benefits such as parking passes, housing, meal cards, etc., including how students gain access to the benefit and when they need to start the process so each benefit is in place when the rotation starts.
- A brief statement regarding accommodations for students with disabilities. Although it's rare, students with disabilities occasionally come through pharmacy programs and must let you know up front if they have specific needs. A statement in the syllabus serves as a reminder to the student, and it documents that you asked for notification.

- A "frequently asked questions" section, which you can add to as the rotation develops.
- Sample calendar, which is discussed in more detail below. Including a calendar as an addendum to your syllabus really helps students hit the ground running on the first day.

Orientation

Orientation is probably your first face-to-face contact with the student. As the saying goes, "You never get a second chance to make a good first impression," which is true for both you and the student.

Make the orientation a formal process that is planned in advance and carried out like any other important event. Time constraints and conflicting demands sometimes lead to informality in orientations. The pitfalls associated with failing to plan and schedule a formal orientation can be summed up by these questions:

- Will the orientation actually happen? When?
- Will you remember to cover everything that's important for the student to know?
- Will the student remember the information you covered?
- Will your understandings match regarding things the student needs to know and do for the rotation to unfold smoothly?
- Are misunderstandings likely, and will they lead to unhappiness?

> Make the orientation a formal process that is planned in advance and carried out like any other important event.

Providing a formalized orientation leads to:

- Clear communication and a solid foundation of information.
- Clear understanding of
  - The practice site and the organization it is part of.
  - Staff duties.
  - Overall expectations.
- Clear and appropriate time frames for each part of the orientation, rather than rushing through.

Initial Contact

The form of your first contact with your student will depend on the college's instructions to its students. At the college where I direct experiential education, I ask students to make initial contact via email and to include a copy of their curriculum vitae (CV).

Preceptors should prepare a document to send by return email as a response, which includes:

- Directions for anything you want students to accomplish before the first day.
- Specific instructions from Human Resources (HR) that students must comply with before arriving on site.
- A copy of the syllabus.
- A plan for the first day that covers the "where, when, and how" of the experience:

  o Where
    - Directions
    - Parking
    - Access to the building
  o When
    - First day start time
    - Normal start time
  o How
    - Preparation
    - Readings and refreshers
    - Key points regarding the syllabus
    - CV (reminder to send a copy to the preceptor if this hasn't been done already)
    - Dress and identification
    - Contact information
    - Clearances and HR requirements

This is not a comprehensive list; other items specific to your site may need to be included. Take the time to construct this document carefully, because you will use it again and again.

First Day

Prepare a detailed plan to kick off the rotation's first day on a positive note—a sort of "day-one syllabus" the student can refer to. As noted above, the first day should be devoted to a formal orientation.

In my opinion, the best orientations are carried out by preceptors themselves. But if you decide to distribute the orientation workload, carve out one-on-one time with the student on that first day, even if just for a few minutes. Meeting together without distractions can go a long way toward making the student comfortable with you and the site.

Points to Cover

Below are some things to cover during your time with the student. Although most are included in the syllabus or in your correspondence, repeating them in person helps to reinforce key information.

- Review course objectives and evaluation criteria.
- Explain expectations for the student's dress and grooming.
- Tour the site, point out particularly important places in the site layout, and introduce the student to the team and employees.
- Provide an overview of other personnel with whom the student will be working, and supply necessary contact information.
- Review computer accesses and uses.
- Discuss expectations for what the student will be doing hourly, daily, weekly, and during the overall experience.
- Go over specific assignments that may require detailed instruction.
- Review the calendar.

Consider having other people conduct specific parts of the orientation, such as HR representatives or members of your staff. This not only helps you use your time efficiently, but introduces students to other personnel who can answer questions. If you are the only person they know, students will come to you for everything.

If time on the first day is a problem for everyone, consider a self-directed orientation, which takes a bit of setup but can be a very good way to structure the day and get the student actively involved. Options include scheduling a series of appointments for the student to attend or creating a scavenger hunt or exploration game that goes something like this: "Find a person named Shirley in room 1001 of the hospital. Learn what charity event she organizes for the hospital. While you are there, get your name badge made." Kind of cheesy, but effective.

You can also segment the orientation into small pieces over the first few days of the rotation. If you choose this route, make sure the first segment contains the essentials.

I've also known preceptors to schedule time with students the day before a rotation. Finding free time on the first day can be difficult, particularly in community practice settings where the rotation starts on the first Monday of the month. Having the student meet with you on Sunday afternoon or evening may make for a far better orientation.

Facts to Learn

The orientation is not just for students; it is also for *you*. You will need to probe the following questions:

- What is their background?
- What do they know already?
- What skills do they have?
- What do they want to learn?
- How can you get in touch with them?

> Providing the first assignment as the last part of your formal orientation is an excellent lead-in to the actual rotation.

Learning the answers helps you understand what they want out of the experience and how you can tailor the experience to them. It also helps you identify skills they possess, which might allow you to try out a new project or activity that, if successful, becomes a regular part of your rotation.

First Assignment

Providing the first assignment as the last part of your formal orientation, or as a separate piece right after a break, is an excellent lead-in to the actual rotation. It should be specific and introductory, reinforcing items covered in the orientation and designed as a foundation to the regular assignments.

In a community setting, the first assignment might be to pick an over-the-counter (OTC) product line appropriate for the time of year, such as cough and cold, and have students simulate a consult with the front-end manager (after you obtain the manager's permission). This assignment familiarizes students with the OTC aisles, acquaints them with tasks they'll regularly conduct during their time with you, introduces them to store personnel, and helps you assess students' starting capabilities.

Troubleshooting

As with anything that is well planned, the potential always exists for something to go wrong. Common ways that orientations can go awry include:

- **No contact.** If you think you are supposed to have a student and have not heard anything, contact the college. Occasionally, an event in the student's life might prevent him or her from getting in touch with you on schedule. Or the student might simply have forgotten.

- **Late contact.** Unfortunately, late contact can result in delayed starts or a need to reschedule the student, based on HR requirements. For example, if a student does not get in touch with you until a week before the rotation begins, completing a required drug screening may not be possible before the first day. If something like this occurs, you must decide if the rotation can still start on time or with a minor delay. Even if the rotation begins as planned, remember to include the student's late contact when evaluating his or her professionalism.

- **Holidays.** Holiday policies vary according to the site, rotation, and college, so check with your college to find out its policy. I require students to adhere to the holiday policy of the site where they are assigned. If the site is open on a given day and the preceptor is there, students should be, too. It is best to be clear about the holiday policy up front by detailing it in the syllabus or orientation.

- **Communication gaps.** Occasionally, preceptors and students have difficulty getting in touch with each other, whether because of a mistyped phone number or an illness. Whatever the reason, the solution is to turn to the college, which knows you both. For example, if a student is scheduled to begin with you in September and you will be gone for two weeks in August, notify the college so it can inform the student. This prevents the student from wondering why you haven't responded to his or her first contact.

Calendar

If the syllabus is a roadmap for the rotation, the calendar is turn-by-turn directions, providing structure that students dearly crave.

Calendars vary quite a bit in how much detail they offer. Some provide specific times and dates for all activities. Some set aside large blocks of time for possible activities; others combine both approaches. No ideal calendar exists; do what works for you and your rotation.

Start with a blank calendar and plug in events that will or might happen for a typical rotation. Consider the following questions:

- What is going to happen daily?
- What is going to happen weekly?
- What is going to happen occasionally?
- What deadlines need to be noted?

Your first calendar will not be perfect. Over time, you'll end up with a much better version after the first few students tell you what you did wrong.

Several shared calendars found online are useful for planning your calendar, such as Google Calendar and Yahoo! Calendar. Using such tools allows students to start with the document you created and then modify it as activities are added or adjusted during the experience.

Chapter 4

Your First Student— A Unique Opportunity

Precepting your first student is going to be a unique experience. Much of what this book has covered so far gets you ready to launch your rotation, but keep in mind that the tools you prepare for the first day will become more polished as you use them on a regular basis. Being a preceptor is a continual learning process.

A key lesson you'll pick up when working with your first student is that students see things differently than preceptors do. And these different perceptions are an advantage as we work toward our goal of making our experience as educationally valuable as it can possibly be.

Your first student will see possibilities you did not see, because he or she:

- Is a student and you are not.
- Is new to the environment and you are not.
- Knows less than you do about patient care.

The Student "Reality Check"

Once we are out of school, it doesn't take long for us to lose the student perspective. It's helpful to pay attention to the student's view of the way you have designed your experience because it allows you to improve its quality. The student may:

- Look at your plan and tell you it involves too much or too little.
- Ask to do things you did not expect him or her to want to do.
- Ask for more or less training on certain topics or skills.
- Feel more or less comfortable doing certain things than you expected.

You may not like hearing this, but in some ways you need an *alternative* syllabus for your first student: one that has objectives specific to the very first student. Why? Because you will get the best results from students when they know that one of their goals is to help improve the rotation.

Enlist Help in Improving the Rotation

Let your first student know that he or she has additional responsibilities—whether by writing it down (which isn't a bad idea) or saying something along the lines of the following:

"In addition to working toward the goals you've already seen in the syllabus, I want you—as the very first student through this rotation—to actively participate in making this experience better for every student who follows you. I am counting on you to do this, and so are they. Look for new learning opportunities, let me know what they are, and tell me why you are interested in them. Give me feedback about the workload, the value of the assignments, the level of support from me and the other people you'll work with, the value of your interactions with the health care team, and so on. If at any time you are having difficulty or something is not working, please let me know as soon as possible so we can try to find a way to make it work better. We will, at several points, sit down and have a feedback session about the experience itself to make sure things are going right and to see about taking advantage of the opportunities you identify."

> It's helpful to pay attention to the student's view of the way you have designed your experience because it allows you to improve its quality.

Informing students up front how much you are depending on them to improve the rotation can make a big difference in their commitment to offering suggestions. This approach also helps smooth out ahead of time the rough edges that will inevitably occur. In other words, knowing they are part of the development process and have a role to play beyond simply being students will make them feel better about events that don't go perfectly.

With each successive student, the need to actively enlist student help for improving the rotation will diminish. (Here I am referring to whipping your practice experience into shape after it is launched—not to continuous improvement over the long haul, which is covered in Chapter 7.) Most of the big gains in value and quality will be made after the first or second student. Of course, any student can trigger new, wonderful changes, but after your first few students, these improvements will come without your specifically asking for input.

Weigh student input carefully, and use what seems appropriate—but don't feel compelled to change things that will alter the heart of the experience. You shouldn't transform your cardiology rotation into an infectious disease rotation just because of student feedback.

Chapter 5

Integrating Your Student into Practice

Over the years, student feedback has convinced me that experiences in which students are fully integrated into a setting are better than those in which student activities are artificially layered alongside the preceptor's. Shadowing and observation do not hold a candle to immersing students elbow-deep in real work.

Although some readers may disagree, I maintain that if students at your site are not adding to your ability to perform the tasks you perform, then you are not integrating students correctly. Or, as the popular Internet meme goes, "You're doing it wrong."

For years, I've heard that students are a burden, they consume too much of the preceptor's time, they take time away from patient care, and so on. But people who say these things don't end up with "preceptor of the year" awards. And the reason they don't is because they have not bought in to the idea of integrating students into their practice.

If you believe from the start that students at your site are going to contribute in a significant way, they probably will.

Boiled down to the basics, integrating students into your practice site efficiently and effectively involves answering three questions:

- What can the students do during the experience?
- What will the experience look like? In other words, what will be your model for an integrated experience?
- Who can supervise it?

Create and Refine a Task List

To figure out what students can do, hold a brainstorming session with others involved in precepting at your site. List all the tasks that students are capable of performing. Avoid limiting the list in any way. In Chapter 2, you performed this exercise to identify functions that provide opportunities for student learning; here you are applying the same approach to identify specific tasks.

Then pare the list down to tasks that match criteria in the bullets below. Ask yourself:

- Does the task fulfill objectives of the experience?
- Is the task performed only during times when students are not present?
- To what degree is this task needed in the environment?
- How valuable is this task to the patient and the site?
- Who would want to do this task if the student were not here?
- Is it a desirable task?

Link Task Value to Objectives

Obviously, tasks we choose for students should meet objectives of the experience. Less obvious is that we can include tasks because they are valuable to the site and then find ways for the tasks to meet educational objectives—or alter our educational objectives to reflect lessons students will gain from those valuable tasks.

I know that seems backward, because usually objectives lead to activities, but think about it this way.

If:
1. We can provide the best educational experiences when students are fully integrated, and
2. We need to include certain valuable tasks to help with that integration, and
3. The experience becomes better by including those tasks,

Then:
4. It was a mistake to leave out those tasks and the associated objectives in the first place.

Following the logic above, including valuable tasks is a way of correcting a mistake because it allows us to integrate students into the experience, boost our efficiency, accommodate more students each year, and provide an educational opportunity that previously didn't exist, thus improving educational possibilities for all students from that point forward.

Consider Timing and Value of Tasks

As for timing, if a task—or at least, the most educational aspect of it—takes place only when students are not present, you might want to consider removing it from the list. You can also adjust students' hours if a task plays a significant role in helping them meet the experience's objectives, but think it through carefully. Changing hours is not always appropriate.

Not all tasks involve the same level of need, and those that are highly needed are not always educationally valuable. Integrating students into tasks that are both educational and needed is the best approach, but it's not always possible. You have to weigh both aspects.

Tasks that are valuable to the site and to the patient tend to be more valuable to students, because students learn more when they're contributing something real to the site and the team instead of carrying out an artificial activity. Therefore, when explaining tasks to students, be sure to spell out the benefit to the site. Some rotations are set up as a series of highly realistic simulations, and although they may provide some educational value, students see through them quickly and eventually lose interest.

> When explaining tasks to students, be sure to spell out the benefit to the site.

If your site has tasks that no one else wants to do, don't be surprised if students don't want to, either. On the other hand, students are new to the site and might not be there long enough to develop distaste for these tasks. You and your staff should avoid pointing out "undesirable" tasks; the student might actually like doing them—and they are worth including if they bring benefits to the site, to patients, and to students' educational development.

Shape the Experience

After identifying tasks for students to do, you need to answer the question, "What will the experience look like?" or "How will it be modeled?" To integrate students into the experience, you have to design their roles and responsibilities so they are integrated from the start. I suggest that you borrow liberally from other successful sites. Do the following:

- Call the director of experiential education at the university you are working with. If you're working with several universities, call a few.
- Ask for a list of the best rotations that are similar to yours.
- Ask what each of those sites does especially well.
- Get contact information for the sites.
- Call the preceptors and talk to them. Maybe even visit if you possibly can. Some useful questions you can ask include:
  o How do you run your practice experience?
  o How are students integrated into your site?
  o Why is your rotation designed the way it is?

I know that these efforts seem like a huge inconvenience, but consider the time you'll save in the future if you start with a solid plan that builds on the lessons of others.

After gathering expert advice, think about which elements you can implement at your site. Because each site is different, the experience must be tailored —but be sure to keep in mind an important principle that was suggested by Marion Slack and JoLaine Draugalis in their article, "Models for estimating the impact of clerkship students on pharmacy practice sites," published in the *American Journal of Hospital Pharmacy,* February 15, 1994. They looked at the two basic types of preceptor models and found that productivity increases when the student functions as a junior colleague who provides service independently or with limited supervision. Figure 5-1 boils this principle down to a very concise image.

The authors point out that in the non-employee model, the students' activities and how they spend their time depend totally on the preceptor's presence. Therefore, the output of the preceptor's time is not enhanced, or is enhanced in only a limited way, by the student's presence. Thus, if the student is not there, the resources used to supervise the student are diverted to other tasks and very little output is lost. In the employee model, the student acts as a

Figure 5-1 | **Experiential Education Model Effects on Productivity**

Non-employee model: student activities depend on presence of preceptor

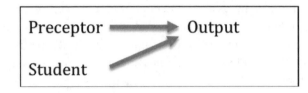

Employee model: student provides service independently or with limited supervision

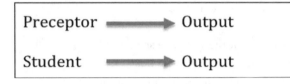

Source: Adapted from Slack MK, Draugalis JR. Models for estimating the impact of clerkship students on pharmacy practice sites. *Am J Hosp Pharm*. February 15, 1994;51(4):525-30.

colleague of lesser experience. He or she provides service independently or with limited supervision while the pharmacist-preceptor carries out other tasks, which means that the loss of a student results in a loss of productivity.

Because pharmacists tend to be "math people," it may help if you look at it this way. If the pharmacist counts as one full-time employee (1.0 FTE) and 0.25 of that FTE goes toward precepting the student, who counts as 0.5 FTE, then the outcome is 1.25 (1.0 − .25 = .75 + 0.5 = 1.25). Although every day won't add up this way, it's what you're shooting for.

Plan Supervisory Roles

Integration involves many things, including planning how the teaching goals mesh with the motivations and desires of other personnel at your site. Delegation and desire must be considered when answering the question, "Who can supervise?"

In Chapter 3, in the section about orientation, I mentioned that students should be informed about who else they'll be working with. An experience can be precepted by a team, which may include pharmacists, residents, other health care providers, technicians, and other ancillary staff. One person must have final say over the experience, but delegating supervision responsibilities to team members can be critical to successfully integrating the student into the site. Delegation also helps avoid burnout among preceptors. For it to work, however, the people taking on supervision responsibility must have the desire to precept, must be accountable for that supervision, and must receive appropriate recognition. Include their names and precepting roles in the syllabus and introduce them at orientation so the student has a clear understanding of each person's responsibilities.

Delegation has the following benefits:

- Creates an environment where students learn from the person who knows each particular area the best.
- Divides the instruction workload so no one is overloaded.
- Exposes the student to a range of professionals and their individual nuances.
- Concentrates learning, depending on the number of students on a site or experience—such as delegating several students to a single faculty member for a discussion group topic in which that person has particular expertise.

Too often, people create silos around their learning experiences. They say "this is *my* student" or "that is *your* student," when in reality we should be saying, "these are *our* students."

It's All About Education

Of course, care needs to be taken. All this talk of integration and "employee" models may cause someone further up the food chain to think that the sole purpose of having students on site is to provide services that don't have to be paid for. In other words, "free labor." This is not the case. Any suggestion of it should be stamped out immediately.

The purpose of having the student on site is *education,* which involves a process of meaningful practice and feedback. When meaningful practice occurs, a benefit can be seen. When a benefit is seen, people at the site are happy and want to take on more students. When more students are placed, more education is possible, and the cycle continues. This is our goal.

Chapter 6
The Importance of Feedback and Evaluation

The other day I was speaking with some senior students who were about to give a presentation at our incoming class's orientation. We were standing outside the auditorium, waiting for our part of the agenda. They asked, "Are you going to give your 'Who do I work for?' speech?"

I was startled that they remembered. And also happy that my words had left an impression. Orientation is so packed with information I'm surprised that they remember anything, much less a short discussion we'd had four years earlier. It made my decision to say the same thing again very easy.

During orientation I typically ask the incoming class, "Who is it you think I work for?" Then I wait for answers. "The university," they sometimes say. Or, "the students." After taking a few replies, I tell them, "I work for the people of the state of Florida. My job is to make sure that one day you don't kill them accidentally, or otherwise. While I very much want each and every one of you to succeed in pharmacy school and become an excellent pharmacist, if I have to choose between your success and their lives...I choose their lives. If you must do something else for the rest of *your* life so they can be better off—then I have done my job."

Melodramatic, yes, but it gets the point across.

Faculty members, even those who volunteer or work part time, have responsibilities I've summarized in the list below.

1. Responsibility to patients.
2. Responsibility to the student.
3. Responsibility to the profession.

In the following pages I'll talk about each, in the context of feedback and evaluation.

Responsibility to Patients

When evaluating students, we must remember that in most cases we are evaluating their ability to care for patients. What happens if they don't do it well? While on rotation they're under supervision, but eventually they won't be.

Most students on advanced pharmacy practice experiences (APPEs) are less than one year from graduating and being responsible for patient care, so by then we have no more leeway. We must evaluate them with honesty. We must evaluate them carefully. We cannot afford to give them the benefit of the doubt. If we do not honor this responsibility, our patients will suffer.

Responsibility to Students

Evaluating students has a threefold purpose. It allows us to:

1. Give positive reinforcement for things they do well.
2. Provide targeted feedback on things they need to improve.
3. If the student is doing poorly enough, remediate so faults and deficiencies can be corrected. In academic settings, remediation involves such steps as repeating courses or taking part in focused tutoring.

Our responsibility for points one and two should not be diminished, but they do not carry the same baggage as point three. That is the hard one, the one most people have trouble with. Telling students they are not currently capable of the work and need remediation is, by nature, a conflict situation. Conflict is not comfortable, and most people avoid it whenever possible. Sometimes it is necessary, however, and this is one of those times.

Consider the situation in which a student performs too poorly to pass the experience. What happens when he passes anyway? The two possibilities are:

1. The student continues to be passed repeatedly without regard for his actual ability. After graduating, he is unable to succeed in the profession or practices so inadequately that he cycles through jobs, harms someone, or ends up at odds with the board of pharmacy.
2. The next person evaluating him wonders how he possibly got past the last experience. His poor performance is spelled out in an evaluation, which puts him in a position to get the remediation he needs—but leaves *him* wondering how he did so well before, but now cannot.

Each scenario is unfair to the student. Preceptors' responsibility is to help students become competent pharmacy practitioners. We cannot do this if we don't evaluate them honestly.

Most colleges have multiple academic markers in place to catch students who are struggling and divert them into a remediation plan. When students perform poorly, getting a low grade signals that remediation is required before they continue in their program—which makes them more, rather than less, likely to eventually succeed.

> Preceptors' responsibility is to help students become competent pharmacy practitioners. We cannot do this if we don't evaluate them honestly.

Typically, students who receive a bad grade will not be "kicked out of school" without a significant prior history of poor performance—in which case, they may be better off in another profession. This attitude may seem harsh, but it's necessary, because our first responsibility is to the patient. We must evaluate students with honesty. We must evaluate them carefully. We cannot afford to give them the benefit of the doubt. If we do not honor this responsibility, our students will suffer.

Responsibility to Our Profession

Before I get too deep into this particular item, let me address an important point. Some might argue that educators are not the gatekeepers for our profession; the gatekeeping responsibility rests with boards of pharmacy, licensing bodies, and testing agencies. I don't agree.

Those agencies certainly play a role, but they cannot be the sole guardians of the public safety. If we wash our hands of our responsibility for education outcomes and willingly give over all obligation to public safety to those agencies, we are no longer acting as professionals. If we don't think of ourselves as gatekeepers, we are effectively stating to the world at large, "Warning! We trained them, but caveat emptor!" Is that really what we want to say about our graduates?

The moment they graduate they are part of our profession—not the moment they are licensed. So when they do poorly, our profession's reputation is sullied—not the reputation of the licensing agencies or testing agencies. If we want our profession to remain strong, it is our responsibility to shape students into the best pharmacists possible before they ever get to those agencies.

Each person you teach becomes part of the next generation of pharmacists. For our profession to remain valued and trusted, we must evaluate students with honesty. We must evaluate them carefully. We cannot afford to give them the benefit of the doubt. If we do not honor this responsibility, our profession will suffer.

Evaluations Essential for Good and Poor Performers

When students believe they are doing well only to find out at the end of the rotation that the preceptor thinks they did poorly, it puts everyone in a bad position. The student is unhappy with the grade, the preceptor is unhappy with all the drama, and the program director is unhappy about mediating between the student and the preceptor. The sad thing is, this scenario is completely avoidable if you follow the four points below.

- Be regular in providing feedback.
- Be comfortable with the evaluation system in place.
- Be consistent in the way you evaluate.
- Be diligent in your documentation.

Regular feedback is not necessarily restricted to what is listed in your syllabus, although it will include those items we mentioned in Chapter 3—observation, performance reports, formal evaluations, and testing. You also need to give feedback at the moment of education, such as:

- Letting students know as soon as they complete a task what they did right and what they can improve on.
- Asking students to self-assess, and using their input as a starting point for a more detailed evaluation of their performance.

Providing feedback regularly throughout the experience helps students stay up to date on their progress. Be positive when warranted, but remember that students who are not doing well need to know. It's tempting to be *too* positive.

Regular feedback should also include formal midpoint evaluations—the same evaluation you complete at the end of their experience with you. Sometimes you might conduct just one midpoint evaluation, but if a student is struggling, conducting several throughout the rotation is helpful to answer for the student, "Where do I stand?" and "How am I doing?"

When students are doing well, evaluations can fall by the wayside. It seems superfluous to tell people over and over that they are doing great. But honestly, positive reinforcement is an excellent way to build the confidence students will need when they become practicing pharmacists. And shortcutting the feedback process for good students prevents preceptors from forming the feedback habit in general. If you don't build the habit, it won't be there to draw on when students are not doing well and need regular, clear guidance about necessary improvements. Conducting periodic evaluations is also important for documentation purposes, even for your star students, as discussed on page 51.

Feedback sessions are not a time for subtlety. I'm not saying, "Don't be nice." I'm saying that there should be no doubt in anyone's mind that feedback has been given and received—and the meaning of the feedback should be clear.

> **Feedback sessions are not a time for subtlety.**

Most pharmacists have been trained in communication techniques that we use regularly to be sure patients understand what we have said to them, yet we don't use these techniques with our students—such as open-ended questions, reflective statements, empathy, and asking for clarification. This discrepancy both amuses and disturbs me. The same skills we employ to interview and counsel patients should be used when providing feedback to students.

Know Your System

As noted in Chapter 3, evaluation systems come in many varieties, from regional approaches to those you develop and use individually. Some groups are working toward standardization, such as the American Association of Colleges of Pharmacy, so that one day pharmacy students everywhere may be evaluated under the same system, but it's a way off.

No matter what evaluation system is employed by the college you are working with, be sure you understand its structure and how it is used for all levels of student performance. I have found that when preceptors struggle with evaluations, it's usually because they have only a superficial understanding of how the system works. They find it easy to fill out an evaluation for a student who does everything right, but when a student is mediocre or poor, they don't know how to make use of the evaluation's system for differentiating performance and skill levels. Most pharmacy students do well, but eventually you'll have one who is not up to par, and you need to be ready.

Avoid Inconsistency

Inconsistency in evaluation systems and grading can take many forms. Avoid inconsistency by understanding the pitfalls discussed below.

Drift

A chronic problem in grading is "drift," which happens when you assign a certain grade to students who perform a certain way, and then compare the next students to them. It's hard not to do this. Over time, the grading drifts up or down rather than staying consistent. If you use one student's performance as your standard rather than an objective, steady reference point, grading will fluctuate.

Level of Experience

The time of year can lead to grading inconsistencies. Should students on their first experience be evaluated differently than those on their fifth? The answer may depend on how the evaluation system is set up. Some systems ask you to evaluate students based on the same standard regardless of how many experiences they have under their belts. Some systems are based on the expectation that preceptors will factor experiences already completed by the student into the evaluation. You must know how your evaluation system works so you use it consistently.

Points for Professionalism

Another source of inconsistency comes from misunderstanding the system's approach for evaluating professionalism. As mentioned in Chapter 3, some systems deduct points on the back end for absenteeism, tardiness, etc. Other systems include professionalism in the grade from the beginning, assigning appropriate weighting so that problems exert a noticeable effect. Inconsistencies can occur when the preceptor believes the system is operating one way, when in fact it is the other.

Document Regularly and Thoroughly

How many times have you heard, "If you did not document it, then it did not happen"? We talk to students about this all the time, and it comes up regularly in staff development sessions. Yet a paucity of documentation is common in student evaluations.

Documenting student evaluations is important for creating a record of what happened in the experience, which is useful when:

- Grade disputes arise.
- A student is struggling and the college needs information to structure the most beneficial remediation plan.
- The college is seeking information to help tailor future educational experiences to maximize benefit for specific students.
- Students want to actively direct their own education. They can say to their next preceptor, "Here is a list of things I have been told to work on."

> Documenting student evaluations is important for creating a record of what happened in the experience.

Whether a student is doing poorly or wonderfully, you should, at the very least, conduct and document a formal midpoint and final evaluation.

Prepare three forms of documentation:

- For your own files.
- For the college.
- For the student.

These can be in hard copy or electronic format. Supplement the evaluation system's output with your own thoughts and impressions. You can also include samples that are representative of the student's quality of work. All three versions of your documentation can be the same, but if any of them are different, most likely it's the one going to the student. The student version should:

- Concentrate on how he or she met or did not meet the objectives of the experience.
- State what the student needs to do in the future to meet the objectives.

Your documentation process and the consistency with which you've applied the evaluation criteria will really pay off if a student disagrees with your evaluation. This may never happen, but if it does, being prepared helps. The student may be wrong. He or she may have good points. At the very least, the student looks at things differently than you do and has a different view of his or her own abilities. Students are entitled to due process in their academic lives, and that process needs to be followed according to the college policies.

Although schools' approaches may differ, the typical path for reviewing a student complaint about an evaluation flows from instructor to course coordinator, department chair, or dean all the way to an institutional student advocate or ombudsman. As soon as a student challenges your evaluation, call the college to find out its policy, if you don't already know it. Someone in charge will spell out specifically what you need to do.

Such situations can be tense, but they are typically not the torture you might imagine. If you follow the policies and stay calm, things will move forward reasonably smoothly. Remember, people at the college have handled similar matters many times, even if you haven't.

Avoid thinking of the situation as a contest between you and the student about who is right. Maintain focus on what's important: patient care and the education of future pharmacists.

Chapter 7

Using Feedback for Continuous Improvement

Four primary sources of information may be useful on a regular basis for improving the practice experience you offer.

- Direct student feedback
- Formal student evaluations
- Feedback from the college
- Peer review

You may not have access to all these options, and they vary in reliability and usability. Let's talk about each in turn.

Direct Student Feedback

In a perfect world, direct feedback from students would be our most productive source of information, but in reality, it's not always reliable. Some students are very willing to give you specific and valuable feedback about how the experience could be improved and what went well. Unfortunately, some students are concerned that what they say will affect their grade, or they are uncomfortable giving constructive criticism to a supervisor. It never hurts to ask for input. Don't be surprised if the feedback you get is not particularly useful, but you may hear something to help you improve.

Although you can gather direct feedback anytime during the experience, the two best times are the formal midpoint and the final evaluation.

Midpoint Feedback

After presenting your midpoint evaluation to the student, say something like this:

"We have talked about how you are doing. Now is a chance for you to let me know how I could do things better for you. I cannot guarantee that we will be able to make the changes you mention, but I am willing to listen and consider what you say. So, what could we change to improve this experience for you?"

After saying this, listen. Do not interrupt except to ask for clarification. If you give the least hint that you are unhappy with the way the interaction is going, you will lose the opportunity to gather this information. Even when something the student says hits a nerve, resist the impulse to respond in the moment.

Later, think about what the student has said. If suggestions were offered that you can implement without changing the direction of the experience or decreasing its quality, consider a trial, at least.

Wrap-Up Feedback

After going over the final evaluation with the student, say something like, "Now that we've completed your evaluation I wanted to give you another opportunity to tell me what we can do to make this experience better. Although I can't change things for *you* at this late date, giving me productive, honest input can help the many students I'll be precepting in the future. I'm sure they'll appreciate it, even if they don't know the suggestions came from you. So, what are your ideas?"

Again, your role is to listen, ask clarifying questions, and thank the student. Later, decide which suggestions you can incorporate and when. You may want to see if other students give the same feedback before you make certain changes. Even ideas that strike you as really good don't have to be implemented immediately.

Sounding Board

During these feedback sessions, feel free to ask students' opinions of ideas that have been put forth previously. For example, "You know, I had John on rotation a couple months back, and he mentioned the same thing. He suggested X. What do you think about that?" While you're engaged with students in a conversation about improvement, you may as well use them as a sounding board for reasonable ideas.

> Feel free to ask students' opinions of ideas that have been put forth previously.

If you are part of a team, don't forget to run feedback and suggestions for changes past the other members. They may have very different views regarding the need and desirability of modifications.

Formal Student Evaluations

Formal student evaluations tend to be more objective and useful than direct student feedback. For each experience, formal evaluations are typically administered by the school, either via paper or electronic questionnaires. At some schools, it's voluntary for students to fill out formal evaluations of the course and instructor; at others, it's mandatory. Although these decisions are beyond your control, it's good to know the requirements of the school you are working with.

The results are presented to you in aggregate form, typically once a year, along with anonymous comments. The information provided from these evaluations can be very valuable. You should concentrate on the following aspects.

Aggregate Question Data

Most evaluations include a series of questions on a Likert scale, in which respondents express their opinion by rating items on a continuum. Schools tend to use standard forms for all courses and experiential education, so each question may not be specifically relevant to your site. Before looking at the responses, read through each question to see if it is applicable to your experience. For example, "The test questions for the course were fair," is irrelevant if you don't administer a test.

Then, on your sheet of aggregate data, assess how much care students took in completing the evaluation by determining whether questions that do not apply to your experience were answered (rather than being marked N/A). If everything matches up appropriately—that is, it appears they answered the questions they should—then you can look for trends.

Most times, the aggregate data sheet will also provide comparisons showing how your experience ranks relative to other experiences similar to yours, which gives you a sense of whether it falls close to the norm. If it doesn't, do not let this information discourage you. Keep in mind that it provides an opportunity for new preceptors like you to grow, and it is not an indictment. Likewise, if your scores fall in line with others or are better than average, it doesn't mean you shouldn't try improvements. Preceptors should react to feedback the way we would like students to react.

Comments Section

Most formalized evaluations give students the opportunity to write comments, which can be an excellent source of specific feedback, depending on the effort the student expends. Much of the time, the comments are generic, such as, "Loved it," "It was great," "I did not like it," or "It sucked"—pretty worthless and, for the most part, to be ignored, unless you receive the same comment consistently. Reading "it sucked" on several evaluations is not a good sign, but unfortunately, it doesn't tell you in what way the experience sucked or how to go about making it suck less.

Although comments are made as anonymous as possible by omitting students' names, it's not that hard to figure out which evaluations might go with which student, especially if you precept only a few a year. This is particularly true if their comments mention specific events, complaints, or compliments that would apply only to a particular student. Even if you can guess who said what, you must at least maintain the illusion of anonymity. You can't go back to students and ask if they made a particular comment and why.

Seeing a certain comment several times without further detail is a sign to get in touch with the director of experiential education at the college. Ask him or her to contact the students independently and gather information about how you could improve the experience.

When the evaluations do contain detailed comments, pay attention to specifics you can use for improvement. For example:

- This APPE needed additional time set aside for X.
- I was expecting X but actually spent more time doing Y.
- I was frustrated by X.
- I was particularly happy with X aspect of this experience.

If someone has taken the time to write it down, it is probably significant to him or her. Likewise, if one person said it, a few others probably thought it. For each such comment, ask yourself the following:

- Is the suggested change in line with the goals and objectives of the experience?
- Would making the change fundamentally reduce the effectiveness of the experience?
- Would the suggested change enhance the experience?

Remember, just because students don't like something or would prefer to do something else doesn't
mean that making changes is the right thing to do.
Likewise, just because the suggestions may lighten
their load does not make them bad suggestions.
Take to heart the comments that will make the
experience better, regardless of whether they make
it harder or easier.

> If one person
> said it, a
> few others
> probably
> thought it.

Here are a few more things to consider when looking at student feedback.

Timing

To preserve students' anonymity, preceptors don't receive evaluation data
until after students are finished with their introductory pharmacy practice
experience or with their entire array of advanced experiences. It could be
a semester or a full year before you get feedback. This delay affects the
evaluations' impact, since the very things brought up in them could have
been identified and resolved in the time that has elapsed since the experience
was completed. To figure out how much value to place on the information,
ask yourself:

- What was going on at that time? If you're not sure when the evaluation
  was filled out, it may contain hints in the comments, such as "the
  preceptor was preoccupied with a Joint Commission inspection."
- What is going on now?
- How much has already changed to address concerns reflected in the
  evaluations?

For example, staffing shortages that caused stress a year ago may show up in
students' comments, but if you've added personnel since then and morale is
high now, there's nothing to fix.

Context

Rotations do not exist in a vacuum. Several factors combine to influence how
they turn out, including you, the student, the site, the patient load, the time
of year, what's going on in your life, and so on. For each piece of feedback,
consider the following questions for insights into what might have shaped the
students' view of the experience. The answers help you determine the value of
the evaluations and which points to focus on the most.

- Who were the students?
- What were the students' goals?
- What was the "team" like?
- What was the patient load?
- What were the students' grades?
- How was the students' experience?

Feedback from the College

Typically, feedback from the college is more intermittent than formal student evaluations are. College feedback usually comes from the two sources discussed below.

Follow-up from Student Feedback

Sometimes the college gets specific feedback from students regarding the experience and, depending on the consistency and volume of the comments, has an obligation to follow up. This sounds bad—and it can be, but it doesn't have to be. The goal of the site, preceptor, and college is to successfully train pharmacy students, so it's best to keep in mind that feedback is in everyone's best interest.

Several years ago I worked with a preceptor whose evaluations involved chronically low ratings. I'd also gotten feedback from individual students who were not particularly happy with the experience. Upon investigation, none of them said they did not learn, but they felt that aspects of the experience were very uncomfortable. I spoke with the preceptor at length about the experience and why he did the things he did. As a result, we determined that nothing should change. In his rotation he chose to emphasize autonomy of action. He expected students to operate without much guidance after the first few days, an approach he spelled out in his objectives. Students had specific goals to meet each day, and he held them accountable.

The students found this autonomy and accountability uncomfortable. The preceptor and I realized that such an experience would probably never receive good evaluations, but that did not stop it from being worthwhile. Students probably would not recognize its value until later in their careers.

Conducting Site Visits

Colleges also conduct regular visits to learning sites to get a hands-on feel for the student experience and to give preceptors the opportunity for face-to-face communication with a college representative. Sometimes this is a formalized process with a very specific format, but other colleges follow a more

> Site visits are an opportunity for exchange and brainstorming.

informal approach. In either case, these visits are not a cause for trepidation; instead they are an opportunity for exchange and brainstorming.

Having a faculty or staff member come to your site and see what you do can lead to new ideas and insights. Preceptors often fail to realize that the college's representative is probably one of the people exposed to the widest variety of pharmacy practices in your state—other than board of pharmacy inspectors. You can pick his or her brain about what is happening elsewhere and learn what others are doing that is working. Take advantage.

Peer Review

Peer review is an excellent source of information about your experience, but can be difficult to set up. In the best-case scenario, someone with no relation-ship to your experience who practices in a similar setting comes to your location and observes for a period of time—the longer, the better. But everyone is busy, and it's tough to find an observer with time to spare.

More likely is finding someone in your practice setting not directly involved with your experience who can dedicate a day or an afternoon to peer review and then give you feedback. A peer reviewer should be experienced enough as a supervisor or preceptor to know which questions to ask and to offer you insight into how things could be improved.

Some colleges may have resources to help with this—anything from an instruction booklet that guides the reviewer through the process to a match-ing system that finds outside reviewers for you. Regardless of how you set it up, it's worth doing every few years for unbiased, productive, professional feedback.

The peer reviewer's mission is to look objectively at the structure of your experience and its implementation. Have the person come on a day when various activities of the experience are showcased so he or she can see as much as possible. The peer reviewer will want to spend time with you as well as your student, observe normal activities, and possibly talk to other members of the health care team. It's hard to avoid modifying what you do while someone is observing, but try to behave naturally so your reviewer can provide the best feedback possible.

> Don't be afraid to embrace new concepts if they will add to the experience.

It's All About Improvement

No matter where your feedback comes from, remember that the goal is improvement. Look at each piece of feedback and see what can be implemented. Keep an open mind. Bounce ideas off colleagues or former students. Don't be afraid to embrace new concepts if they will add to the experience.

Never forget, though, that you are the final arbiter of what will work. If the changes suggested are not going to improve the experience, don't do them.

Chapter 8

Precepting as Art Form

The many articles and books that have been published about precepting are full of great ideas, examples, and methods for teaching students, but one thing they leave out is that teaching is an art.

Merely putting scientific theories and principles into practice about the best way to do this or that does not guarantee a good outcome. Desire, talent, experience, creativity, and responsiveness are important, too. The way precepting is done—the art—is what creates an outcome worth having.

The Photographer-Preceptor

Trying to find a recognizable art form as an analogy, I thought about painting, but realized it's probably not a good choice because painters don't have to be good technically to be well respected for their art. A better analogy might be photography, which takes the photographer, the equipment, the environment, and the subject to make an artistic photograph. If the equipment is bad—a cheap disposable camera, for example—or the subject is bland or the environment is horrible, with bad light and background clutter, a true artist can still turn out an amazing picture.

If we consider ourselves technical preceptors only, we will always be restricted by our tools, our environment, and our subjects. As artist preceptors, we understand that although we may be limited by these things, we can overcome them to achieve wonderful results. So, how do we do that?

Artists see things that others do not see, and they see in ways that others do not. In a like manner, we should look at the experiences we provide with our minds open to new ideas and opportunities. Often, wonderful experiences come from people taking the time to recognize possibilities that others have not seen.

Be Aware

In your site, be constantly aware of what is changing. What is happening that could be adapted for learning or adopted from some other area and applied to your rotation? Look at each change as a way for your students to become more involved. Anytime someone comes to you with a problem, or you hear about a problem, think about how you and your students could help solve it. Even if you can't solve it, exploring options will open up new vistas.

For example, several years ago a community pharmacy preceptor learned about a state program to help elders gain access to drug assistance programs. It was staffed by volunteers who, though dedicated, lacked skills and resources that health care professionals have. He contacted me about getting his students involved with the volunteers and expanding the opportunities to counsel these elders. The students learned firsthand how assistance programs work, while at the same time sharing their knowledge about drugs and drug therapy. The students' contribution was so successful that we duplicated the setup in other cities.

It's easy to find a way to do something and to stick with it, but that approach can lead to boredom and stagnation. You're a better preceptor when you're engaged and enthusiastic. Use new opportunities to refresh your interest in teaching so your motivation does not fall off. The same creativity you apply to solve patients' problems can help you see possibilities in your site.

Sometimes good photographers just happen to be in the right place at the right time with their camera handy.

Be aware of what your colleagues are doing at your site and other sites. What works and what doesn't? Sharing ideas about precepting can lead to exciting possibilities.

In addition to learning about colleagues' successes, finding out what didn't work is helpful because:

- You can avoid wasting time on fruitless efforts.
- You can learn about approaches that may be just right for your setting, even though they didn't pan out elsewhere. Returning to the photography analogy, a good photographer can see a technique used by another and apply it to his or her own art in completely different ways.

Several years ago, a pharmacist just starting her hospital position was hesitant to precept students because she feared her hodgepodge of responsibilities wouldn't provide enough focused work for students each day. She attended our annual preceptor workshop and talked to another preceptor who had taken part in a combination rotation of two four-week periods strung together. For eight weeks the student focused on two somewhat-related areas. This pharmacist realized she could take part in a such an arrangement and contacted a colleague with concerns similar to hers. They two got in touch with me and I helped them work out the details of an eight-week combined rotation. That experience is still going strong.

Pharmacy practices everywhere have commonalities, but they have unique aspects, too. Be aware of what makes your practice special. Find the little things that differentiate it, and accentuate them. You like what you do for a reason, which is reflected in nuances in your practice that you can capitalize on to enhance your learning experience. Sometimes, art focuses not on the main subject, but on some smaller detail picked out and put on display.

I once worked with a preceptor who had a true passion for community service. He spent a great deal of his private time volunteering at clinics for underserved populations and brought his students there to witness that side of health care and his enthusiasm for it. Over time he gave up having students at his practice site and only precepted them in the underserved clinics.

Be aware of your *students*' differences, as well, and let these differences help you direct their learning. Use your students' creativity to help you find new opportunities for them and for the students who follow. Two minds are better than one. Over the course of your years as a preceptor, you will be exposed to hundreds of creative minds. Not taking advantage of them would be a tragedy. The results can be impressive.

One student asked if it would be possible to set up an advanced pharmacy practice experience (APPE) at a youth camp dedicated to diabetic children, where she had volunteered as a counselor. The camp was run by a staff of health professionals—mostly volunteers—and operated throughout the summer, with different weeks dedicated to different age ranges. I had never done anything like this before, but it sounded interesting. After some investigation and planning, we eventually implemented the APPE, and students have participated every summer. It is one of the most immersive patient care experiences we provide, giving students 24-hour exposure to patients. The students consider it "life-changing," and the camp organizers absolutely love our students' involvement. The synergy is amazing. Yet it would not have happened had that student not come to me with the idea.

Don't Be Afraid

Don't be afraid to take risks. Involve students in new services and projects. Sometimes they will work out, and sometimes they won't. But if you assume they won't work without trying them, you'll miss out on the possibility of success.

Certainly any new venture needs to be monitored, but sometimes new ideas don't hit the implementation phase because no one is willing to pull the trigger. In strategic planning circles you hear talk of guarding against "ready, fire, aim." In principle, "aim" is good, but it really does need to be followed by "fire." Too often, people operate on the "ready, aim, aim, aim, aim some more, and maybe we should go back to ready?" principle. How many beautiful pictures would have been missed if the person behind the lens chose not to click the shutter?

Don't be afraid to care. Artists have passion. Preceptors can have it, too. When things go well with a student, we should be happy for them and for us. When things go poorly, we should be disappointed for them and for us. Sometimes we shy away from caring about our charges because we're trying to insulate ourselves from disappointments and troubling times. It evens out the emotions, but also cuts us off from the joy. Artists embrace the good with the bad. Rejoice in the good. Embrace the value of the bad in the way it helps you forge a better future.

According to the Art

If I've stretched the artist analogy too far, thank you for your patience. My point is that we're immersed in a profession that is based in hard fact and science. It is easy for us to forget our creative side.

Think back to the teachers you learned the most from. Were they technically proficient? Yes, probably so. Were they also creative in the way they delivered information and directed your learning? Also, probably so. Think about the way they said things, the style with which they interacted with students, the caring they put into designing opportunities. These are the artists you can look to for inspiration. Learn from their examples and become an artist yourself.

Secundum artem, "according to the art," applies to more than compounding.

Chapter 9

Overcoming Student Problems— Laying the Groundwork

Most students are not going to have problems. However, as I tell my preceptors, "There is a bell curve everywhere. Sometimes you just hit the wrong slice." Over the years, I've discovered that most questions from preceptors have to do with student problems.

This chapter gives a basic framework through which to view and address student problems. It's followed by eight case studies that are composites of actual incidents I've encountered over the years.

Predicting which students will have problems is difficult. Certainly, students who struggle with the didactic portion of their curriculum may also struggle with the experiential component, but the two are not always connected. I have seen students blossom once they hit their clinical training. Suddenly, it all makes sense to them. I have also seen students do well in their coursework only to do poorly in the practice environment.

Some students cause concern for reasons that are hard to define, such as being socially awkward, eccentric, or high maintenance. Their professors think, "Oh boy, we are going to deal with problems from *this* one all year." Sometimes their prediction is true, but other times, these students do just fine.

Because the number of students who have a problem while on rotation is so low, it could be years before you have to deal with one. If you're unlucky, however, you could end up with a string of them. The general guidance in this chapter, along with the case studies, should help you deal with specific issues in a professional and productive way.

Focus on Patients

"Are patients in danger?" is the first question you should ask yourself when faced with a student problem. I learned that many years ago from my department chair at the time, David Angaran, and this question guides me constantly in my role as experiential director. If the answer is "yes," your only responsible action as a preceptor is to pull the student off patient care duties until a resolution is found.

> "Are patients in danger?" is the first question you should ask yourself when faced with a student problem.

In general, quality of patient care should be the yardstick that preceptors use to determine if a student's behaviors are appropriate for the setting. When students have good patient care as the focus of their goals, good education will naturally follow.

I drew Figures 9-1 and 9-2 to show my students the right and wrong "world view" of clinical training. If they see themselves at the center, with patient care and their education revolving around them, they need to readjust their perspective. Soon they will be practicing pharmacists and will be unable to shirk their patient care responsibilities or pass them off to someone else.

Figure 9-1 |

**The Wrong World View
for Pharmacists**

Figure 9-2 |

**The Right World View
for Pharmacists**

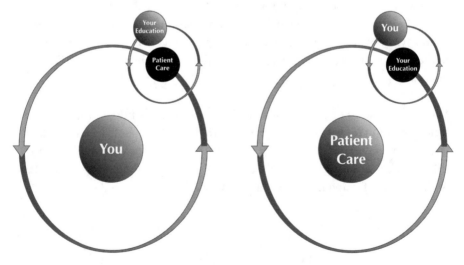

To identify a person's view, think about whether he or she needs to be reminded to handle a personal matter, such as doctors' appointments, oil changes, or even eating lunch. People who are focused on patient care, as in Figure 9-2, sometimes forget to take care of themselves. If, on the other hand, he or she regularly wants to be released from patient care duties or has to be reminded of them, the person probably holds the view shown in Figure 9-1 and sees patient care as something that happens "when I get to it."

Motivation

Although I will not get too deep into the theories of motivation, it's important to remember the two types, intrinsic and extrinsic, and to understand what you do and do not have control over.

Every student is motivated by both types to some degree. Table 9-1 gives examples.

Table 9-1 | **Examples of Students' Intrinsic and Extrinsic Motivation**

Intrinsic	Extrinsic
A desire to do well	Grades
A desire to help others	Future monetary goals
A desire to compete with others	Approval from parents or others
An interest in the area of practice	

In general, preceptors can only *influence* intrinsic motivation factors, but may be able to directly *affect* extrinsic ones. Ways to exert influence could include:

- Challenging students to do well in an area that does not particularly interest them.
- Pointing out how things they are doing might apply to a different area of practice that *does* interest them.
- Illustrating the impact they are having on patient care in their current assignment and how the assignment relates to their future career plans.

Ways to have direct effects could include trying to correct poor behavior by:

- Lowering their grade.

- Postponing their graduation date, which also causes them to lose income, because their entry into practice will be delayed.

Of course, positive reinforcement is better than negative reinforcement, but when a student's goal is to become a health care professional, poor performance cannot be tolerated, and remediation may be necessary.

Locus of Control

The concept of locus of control was developed by psychologist Julian Rotter in the 1950s and 1960s to describe the extent to which individuals believe they can control events that affect them.

- People with an external locus of control feel that outside forces direct or control their life. They tend to blame those forces when things go poorly and give credit to them when things go right.

- People with an internal locus of control see a connection between the outcomes in their life and the things they do.

The locus of control personality trait is not "either/or"; it falls on a continuum and may vary depending on events. Problems can arise on either end of the continuum. For example, student pharmacists with a strong internal locus of control may beat themselves up when things go wrong because they believe they are entirely to blame.

Taking Responsibility for Failures

Pharmacy students tend to be bright and to do well academically, which, of course, is how they made it into pharmacy school. Not particularly startling information, I know. They expect to continue to excel—which can be unrealistic as they progress through pharmacy school. Pharmacy programs are harder than high school and undergraduate studies, so students who succeeded before with little effort may struggle when they hit pharmacy school.

Some will react to pharmacy school's challenges by pushing themselves harder and picking up the study skills necessary to do better. Others won't see their poor performance as their problem, but rather, as someone else's. They may see themselves as persecuted, abandoned, or unlucky, which interferes with their ability to improve.

Just as adjusting to pharmacy school can be hard, some students may flounder when jumping from standard coursework to practice-based learning in experiential rotations. And some may refuse to take responsibility for their failures, putting the blame elsewhere.

> Some students may flounder when jumping from standard coursework to practice-based learning.

- They may blame their previous education. *"They never taught us that."*
- They may blame the preceptor. *"You never told me I should know that."*
- They may blame outside influences. *"My dog ate my homework."*

Some of these reasons could actually be true, but most of the time the problem is that students do not understand their own shortcomings and are unwilling to accept that they are the source of their poor performance.

The Path of Least Discomfort

Although we always hope that our students want to be challenged and to push themselves to learn and improve, it's not always the case. It may sound cynical, but I strongly believe that without very specific reasons to do otherwise, humans will follow the path of least resistance. We avoid what makes us uncomfortable and gravitate to what makes us happy.

This tendency is not necessarily bad. For example, when we're young it keeps us from touching a hot stove twice. But as we mature, it can be the basis for procrastination and other avoidance behaviors. Why do we put off our tax returns until the last minute? Why don't we visit Aunt Edna? Why do our student evaluations take longer than they should to complete? Why don't we like to go to the dentist?

We avoid certain things in the hope that they'll go away and we'll never have to do them or that someone will do them for us. Eventually, the discomfort of not doing them and facing the consequences takes precedence, and we do what needs to be done.

With students, offer the opportunity to do something the easy way or the hard way and they'll do a quick risk/benefit analysis to determine which path pays off the most while making them the least uncomfortable. If the path is hard enough, and the reward not high enough, students will choose the easy way. With this in mind, you can identify the activities in your rotation that might lead to avoidance and procrastination. Modify the reward system so the risk/benefit ratio makes it worth doing, and doing on time.

Unintended Consequences

As an experiential programs director, I've had many opportunities to see both good and bad outcomes of preceptor–student interactions. Everything we do while precepting students has the potential to affect their behavior. Sometimes the changes are not what we want or expect; they are unintended.

For example, a style of teaching commonly used in medical and pharmacy education—the question and answer session—can bring unintended consequences. The following story may seem like a digression, but bear with me.

Alexander Karelin, a massive Russian dominating the heavyweight divisions of world Greco-Roman wrestling from the late 1980s to 2000, was unbeaten for 13 years. He's a highly educated man, with a PhD in physical education, and no one ever scored points against him. His domination of the sport was so complete that his competition actually stopped trying.

His success hinged primarily on his ability to do a reverse lift, which other heavyweight wrestlers could not do, although it's common in the lower weight classes. In this maneuver, the wrestler grabs his opponent around the waist from the back, physically picks him up, and tosses him over the wrestler's shoulder onto the mat. Most of the time, the opponent falls on his head and neck, which is very painful—especially when you weigh 290 pounds—and is embarrassing in the wrestling world.

Over time, his opponents began changing their behavior. Knowing that inevitably they were going to be thrown on their heads and lose, they started choosing the moment that they would lose. Just before Karelin executed his reverse lift, they rolled over and got pinned to save themselves pain and humiliation. Thus, for several years in world competition, including the Olympics, the gold medal was essentially predetermined to be Karelin's, and everyone else played for silver. This lasted until the 2000 Olympics, when the USA's Roulon Gardner stunned the wrestling world with his victory over Karelin.

So, what's the link to the concept of unintended consequences in experiential education? As teachers, we have a significant advantage over students in both knowledge and power—what I call a "knowledge gradient" and a "power gradient." Knowledge in that we actually know more than they do, and power because we have control over their progress through the curriculum.

For us to function as preceptors and mentors, these gradients are necessary and useful. We couldn't teach if we didn't know something students don't know, and we couldn't direct them through a curriculum if we had no power over their actions. However, these gradients can be abused. If we use them to "beat down" the student intellectually, we can induce behaviors in them that may affect their ability to learn from that point forward. The unintended consequence may be that they stop trying to excel, and instead try only to survive, just like Karelin's opponents. We don't want our students to be in this position. We are not in competition with them.

So, in the classic Q&A session, the preceptor poses questions, the student answers correctly, and the preceptor progresses to more difficult questions. Eventually the student gets one wrong or says, "I don't know." A typical scenario is for the preceptor to stop lobbing questions and launch into a mini-lecture on whatever topic the student didn't know. After enduring several difficult sessions like this, the student starts saying "I don't know" earlier and earlier. He's learned how to avoid the pain. If the result is going to be inevitable failure, why wait for it to unfold? This is the unintended consequence.

I'm not dismissing Q&A sessions as an educational methodology. They are valuable because they:

- Put students in a position to answer questions they may be asked when they are practicing pharmacists.
- Help students gain confidence in their abilities.
- Promote students' ability to advocate for patients by providing opinions based on the evidence and supporting their stance.
- Challenge students to use analysis and other high-order thinking skills.
- Allow real-time feedback in which the instructor can tailor learning.

However, none of this can happen if a student says "I don't know." Preceptors must gauge how far they can push so that the Q&A session maintains its value. Some students feel challenged and invigorated by Q&As. The ones we need to worry about, however, are those who lack confidence or whose fear of failure contributes to poor performance. Pay attention to body language that shows frustration or defeat, such as slumped shoulders, downcast eyes, leaning back, or crossed arms. Students who exhibit such body language may need some special care to build their confidence.

Tips for avoiding unintended consequences in Q&As include:

- When a student fails at a question or takes too long to answer, avoid the temptation to rescue. Silence is very uncomfortable, and students believe they can outlast you. Instead of supplying the right answer, pose questions that tap more commonly known information or that require less detailed responses. When students answer correctly, give them positive feedback and move down the path toward the failed question, helping them link information until they craft the correct response.

- Vary the end point of the session or the stream of questions. Make sure the last question is not always one for which the student gave a wrong answer. Sometimes, even if another question logically follows, leaving it for another session—so students end with a correct answer—helps their confidence. You can also wrap up by preparing the student for another Q&A session with a proposed question. "That's correct. Very nice! Now, tomorrow I am going to ask you about X, so make sure you are ready." If the question and answer session always ends in a failure, you may unintentionally reinforce negative feelings.

- If a student clearly seems distressed during a Q&A session, continuing may be counterproductive. However, you don't want to reinforce the behavior of displaying distress to avoid the session completely. Instead, stop and calmly let the student know that his knowledge on that subject will be checked later, and schedule the day and time so he can prepare. When the session arrives, let him start by giving an overview of the topic, which may help create a relaxed atmosphere. Then launch into specific questions.

Q&As are just one example of a situation in which unintended consequences can arise. Unintended consequences can crop up anywhere when preceptors interact with students. Watch for patterns in students' responses, and use behavior modification to bring about better educational outcomes.

Table 9-2 | Today's Generations

	Veterans (Born 1925 to 1945)	Baby Boomers (Born 1946 to 1960)	Generation X or Xers (Born 1961 to 1980)	Millennials or Generation Nexters (Born 1981 to 2000)	Generation Z (Born 2001 to the present)
Basic Values and Traits	- Hard work - Dedication - Sacrifice - Honor - Discipline - Conformity	- Optimism - Team orientation - Involvement - Personal gratification - Personal growth - Loyalty - Career driven - Challenge and choice	- Diversity - Pragmatism - Techno-literacy - Fun and informality - Self-reliance - Fiercely independent - Multitask masters - Work/life balance	- Realism - Feel civic duty - Confident - Achievement oriented - Extreme fun - Respect for diversity - Communal	- Still being formed and defined

Source: Adapted from Askew JP. *From Student to Pharmacist: Making the Transition.* Washington, D.C.: American Pharmacists Association; 2010: 109–10.

Generational Issues

The generation that students come from affects how they perceive the world and the ways they prefer to interact, learn, and solve problems. It's outside the scope of this book to go into the research that has been conducted on generational differences, but reading about it and adjusting your teaching approach for generational styles (summarized in Table 9-2) can be very helpful.

Keep in mind the following when considering generational traits and attitudes.

- The information is based on generalities. Each student should be looked at as an individual. Just because someone is a particular age does not mean that he or she will react the same way as his or her peers. Don't make assumptions. Use the generational information for guidance, not as a master plan. Learn from the student and react appropriately.

- Whether a person falls into one generational category or another does not change our goals for them. At the end of their rotation they all need to know the same things, have the skills to perform the same tasks, have the proper attitude, and do things for the right reasons. How they reach those goals might differ, but the goals do not. At the end of the day they have to be able to take care of patients effectively.

Incentives and Disincentives

I am no psychologist, but my experience has taught me that in general, people change their behavior because of incentives and disincentives. Understanding a student's motivation, locus of control, generational background, and so on can help you figure out which incentives or disincentives may influence a student's behavior.

> In general, people change their behavior because of incentives and disincentives.

Although you can influence behavior, beliefs are not so easily altered. Beliefs, which are held internally, change over time as a person gains life experience and maturity. Preceptors are part of this life experience, so students' contact with us may alter their beliefs, but not because we applied incentives or disincentives. "Think this way or else" doesn't work; neither does, "Think this way and get a cookie." It's important to understand the role that incentives and disincentives can play, as well as their limitations, when dealing with student problems.

Now, to the cases!

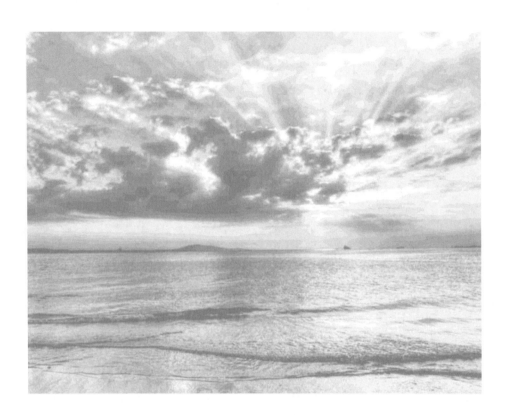

Case
Studies

Case 1

Motivation

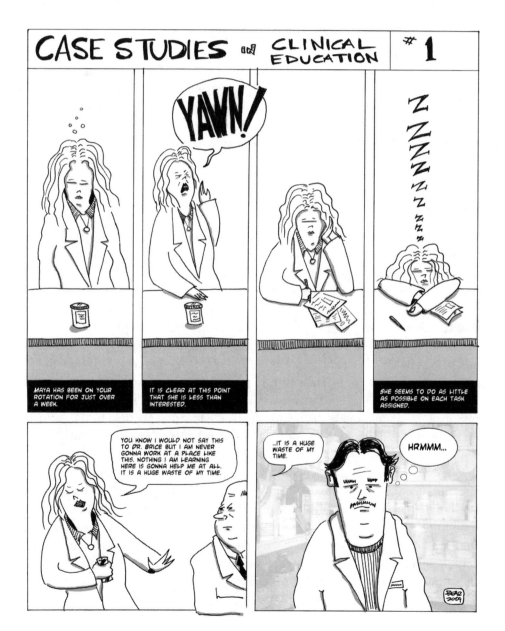

In the case in the illustration, Maya, the student, is clearly not interested in the area she's assigned to. Students have preconceived notions about what kind of practice they are interested in that come from previous experiences, things they've heard, and so on. However, it's too early in their career for them to really know what will suit them. As far as I can tell, their lack of interest has nothing to do with the particular site or area of practice.

Sometimes preceptors get upset when they discover that students are not interested in their practice area. They take it personally or feel that their type of practice is being picked on. "Why do I always get these students who have no interest in learning about [insert practice area here]?" is a question I hear from preceptors in hospitals, community pharmacies, and everywhere in between. Although I'm not going to say, "You shouldn't feel that way," I think preceptors tend to take students' lack of interest in a particular career path too much to heart.

Plans Change

While in school, students regularly change their future plans. Even right before graduation many students remain uncertain about where they are going to practice. They may think their minds are made up, but the truth is, many will change their minds multiple times.

Those of us who have already graduated know that where people start in practice is often not where they end up. "End up" is even a misnomer, considering how often pharmacists change positions and alter their careers. So although a practice area may not interest certain students at the moment, the reality is that they don't know. And we *know* that they don't know, so preceptors' responsibility is to provide them with the best education possible in the setting they're in at the moment, regardless of students' beliefs about its benefits.

Remember, we are training generalists, not specialists. Even if I have a metaphysical certainty—the highest degree of certainty possible for humans to attain—that after graduation a student will practice in a specific area, I must train him or her as a generalist, in accordance with the degree that will be conferred. In PharmD programs, experiential education is supposed to provide both depth *and* breadth of practice. Breadth sometimes means opening up areas that students might not have considered otherwise. If we did not do this, how would they ever be exposed to new things?

Every year, students come to me and say, "You know, I didn't really want that experience, but now that I've had it, I'm considering going into [insert practice area] after I graduate." If we sent students only to places they already wanted to go, this wouldn't happen—and there's no guarantee they'd be motivated once they got to the places they already wanted to go.

Although sending an unmotivated student home may be an option, it should be our last recourse. What other things can we do?

Possible Approaches

Let's think about Maya's current motivation. What did we discover about her during orientation that might help? What are her current and future plans? What kinds of pharmacy practice has she enjoyed to date? This information can help us understand her intrinsic motivation and how we might influence it, as discussed in Chapter 9.

If we don't know these things, we need to find them out through open and direct communication. Talk to Maya about her interests, and perhaps give her an assignment that gives her time to think and formulate better answers. Your conversation might go something like this:

> "Maya, I get the impression that this area of practice is not of particu-lar interest to you. Not everyone who comes through this experience will enjoy it the same way I do, but I would like for all my students to get something out of it that benefits them in the future.
>
> With that in mind, I have an assignment for you. I want you to come in tomorrow with a list that answers the following questions:
>
> - So far, what experiences in pharmacy have really sparked your interest?
> - Where do you plan to practice pharmacy after you graduate?
> - What kinds of pharmacy practice have you heard or read about that sound interesting, but you've never had a chance to see or experience them?
> - Up to this point, what have you found most and least interesting in this experience?
>
> I promise I'll review the list and see how to match up your interests and the site's opportunities, if you promise to work with me to do the

same. We'll have to make sure that the core parts of this experience are covered, but we will try to get creative in the parts where we have flexibility."

Any student who really wants to learn and improve will jump at this opportunity. Good students don't want to be uninterested and bored. If Maya doesn't respond to such a conversation, however, maybe she is just trying to get through the rotation and doesn't want to expend the effort to improve her opportunities, in which case you must use extrinsic motivators, which we'll discuss further on page 82.

Tap the Continuum of Care

Let's assume Maya is willing to try to improve the situation. Act as soon as possible on the information you gained about her interests and plans. Any delay could cause her to lose trust in the process. To tailor your efforts to help with her motivation, ask yourself these questions:

- How does my practice overlap with the things she has interest in or wants to do?
- What tasks or skills used in the practice areas she likes are also used in our practice area?
- Where are the intersections between the patients in my setting and the patients in the setting she is interested in?

Let's say that your experience is based in a hospital inpatient setting and Maya's interest is in home care. An overlap occurs in the time between discharge and the time when home care is in place. Look into exercises focusing on patients who will end up in the home care setting.

If your experience is in community pharmacy and Maya is interested in pain management, create focused exercises in which she develops educational information that can be used with patients in the community setting to teach them about over-the-counter options, ways to manage severe pain, and so on.

If your experience is in critical care and Maya's primary interest is nuclear pharmacy, organize time for her to spend with the radiologist to see how the critical care setting uses nuclear pharmacy drugs.

Remember, patient care is a continuum. Connections exist everywhere from one patient care area to another. Students often don't see this, but you can. Use this.

The options described above can go a long way toward improving the situation for both you and the student. They will not suddenly change her mind about what she likes or dislikes, but they can make the experience more pleasant and produce a better educational outcome. If igniting her interest in certain aspects of the rotation improves her mood, she may see the entire experience in a better light.

Notice, however, that in the sample conversation above, the preceptor said, *"We'll have to make sure that the core parts of this experience are covered."* You can't change the base objectives of an experience just to accommodate a student's level of motivation. It is, after all, part of the curriculum—a curriculum designed to produce pharmacists. Student input is helpful, but the final responsibility for the content is with the faculty.

When Intrinsic Motivators Fail

So what happens if Maya doesn't respond to your efforts to influence her intrinsic motivation? She's not interested and nothing is going to change that. Although some students may have this mindset, it's uncommon and isn't necessarily their baseline: other factors could place them in a "just wanna get through this" mode.

Burnout can happen during clinical experiences. Significant life events can occur that spike behavior in a student that's out of character for her. We all must remember that just because a student is unmotivated now does not necessarily mean she has always been unmotivated. Let's be careful not to assign a pattern to a person and give up on him or her when we have only one point of data.

When students do not respond to intrinsic motivators, contact the college to ask for advice, policies that outline appropriate extrinsic motivators, and documentation procedures so you have written backup about the issues you are dealing with and the strategies you have tried. The mere fact that students know the college has been informed can be enough to make them understand the seriousness of the situation. Sometimes students can be blissfully unaware of just how close to the precipice they are.

The college should be able to let you know if this is a new issue with the student or an ongoing pattern. You can also send correspondence to the student that is openly cc'd to a college representative.

Extrinsic Motivators

Regardless of the reasons behind Maya's lackluster interest, sometimes we need to delve into extrinsic motivations, such as those listed in Chapter 9, page 67. Not all will work on every student, such as grades, for example. Students are well aware of the requirements of their program. If they know they are unlikely to fail the rotation, and that earning less than an A will still allow them to progress toward graduation, they may not be motivated to change their behavior when confronted with the possibility of a lower grade.

Even so, it's worth starting with grades when resorting to external motivators. Have a direct, pointed conversation. Tell Maya what you've observed and ask for her take on it. You might say something like this:

> "Maya, from my perspective it seems you are not very interested in what is available for you to learn here. [Provide specific examples of the evidence of this lack of interest.] This is frustrating. What are your thoughts?"

Her response could take you in several directions. Do not allow yourself to be drawn into a defensive argument. Concentrate on observable facts and, if necessary, your feelings on the subject, which are two things that are not hers to argue. No matter where the conversation leads, come back to a review of the experience's requirements. Wrap up with what you expect from her and the consequences of not meeting those expectations.

> "Maya, although I don't necessarily agree with your take on things, I think we should move ahead. What that means is, for this experience, you are required to do the following: [list the requirements in detail]. Failure to meet these requirements will result in the following grade penalties [list the grade penalties]."

Document the conversation in the form of a written contract on letterhead that spells out expectations, specific goals for Maya to accomplish, and consequences, so there can be no doubt. Put signature lines at the bottom for both of you, and be sure that you and Maya sign off on it. The more formal the process, the better.

Hold firm to what you've put in the contract. It's not good for your future as a preceptor if you can be manipulated into repeatedly adjusting deadlines and goals. If word gets out that you do not stick to your guns, other students may take advantage. Be careful that you are the one training students and not the other way around.

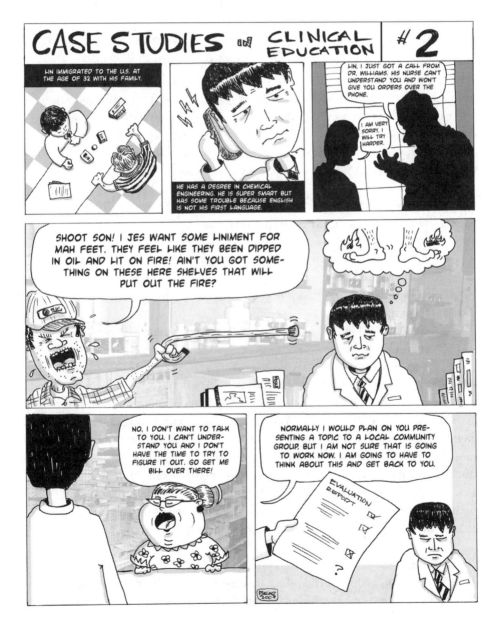

One of the wonderful things about the United States is that it's a melting pot of cultures and ethnic groups. Some parts of the country are more diverse than others, but in general, pharmacy students and patients have a mix of backgrounds. In the example on page 85, Lin, the student, has language deficits. Lin comes from the Pacific Rim and is just like anyone for whom English is a second language and who struggles with language during pharmacy school.

Patient Care First

Let's remind ourselves of our responsibilities. Patient care first. How can a student's poor language skills affect patient care? Lin, like any student in a practice environment, must be able to communicate accurate information to other health professionals and patients, and must be able to understand what they say to him. Even when all parties speak the language well—with full command of vocabulary and grammar—accents and dialects can interfere with comprehension and cause communication breakdowns.

In Florida, where I'm located, students and patients have many different backgrounds, leading to such combinations as:

- Student with Spanish as a first language and patient with a deep southern rural accent.
- Student with Korean as a first language and patient with a Creole background.
- Student with Polish as a first language and patient who is a Mexican migrant worker.

Misinterpreting an order from a doctor or having patients misinterpret directions for their medications can lead to severe, if not fatal, problems. Given the risks, we must consider very carefully whether a student with a language deficit, including an accent so strong that listeners cannot understand him or her, should be in a patient care area. It may seem harsh, because it's not as if such students are not trying. Aren't we penalizing them for something beyond their control? That's not our intent, but if the students' language skills present a danger, we must remove them from the practice environment or at least change their duties to avoid putting patients at risk.

Yes, limiting students' exposure to patients also limits their education, but if you cannot do one without the other, it's best to put their education on hold until the situation is corrected, as explored later in this case discussion.

It's a difficult assessment, and it's entirely up to you. Feel free to contact the college for guidance, but remember that, in the end, you are the person responsible for protecting your patients.

How We Got Here

What can we do about Lin's situation? Before we look at options, let's look at how we got here. More than likely, the root of this problem was in place well before Lin ever arrived at the rotation. Perhaps it started during the college of pharmacy admission process. Admission committees owe it to students to turn them away if they are not likely to be successful. Students with poor language skills should be directed to remediation before being admitted to a college of pharmacy, but this does not always happen.

The standardized tests for assessing speaking skills have limits when it comes to examining whether a student's English is up to the level needed in health care settings. Interviews can be helpful and are now required, but applicants to colleges of pharmacy are very motivated people. If they have a general sense of the questions to be asked, they can prepare well enough to squeak by in an interview. It's not that they are trying to deceive; they are simply unaware of the problems their language skills will eventually cause. They see the barriers to entering pharmacy school as things to overcome, not requirements to meet.

Once students are in pharmacy school, assignments in which they have to communicate are often set up in such a way that they can prepare themselves well enough to get by. Often, it's not until they're placed in a practice environment, where every situation is different and spontaneous, that their deficits are truly identified.

The ideal solution is to help such students early, as discussed at the end of this case, but they must be willing, and often they find the process of receiving extra help with their language skills very uncomfortable.

A few years ago I had a student of nontraditional age who had met her husband in South America and moved to the U.S. with him. In our pharmacy program she struggled with language issues, and was especially uncomfortable on the phone, which showed up in her introductory pharmacy practice experience (IPPE) in a community pharmacy. When we talked about this, she confided that she does not use the phone at home and lets her husband handle all phone conversations. Not until her IPPE forced her to take stock of her deficit did she decide to work on it—a classic example of people avoiding things that make them uncomfortable, while, in the meantime, their problem grows worse.

Each year at orientation for our first-year pharmacy class, I hold a voluntary meeting with those who identify themselves as speaking English as a second language. I explain that I want them to succeed, and to do that, they must be comfortable with English because I don't have experiential practice sites in their first language. Then we talk about how they can prepare:

- Speak English at home.
- Get English-speaking roommates so they're forced to speak English.
- Let the college know immediately if they are having problems, before their progression in school is affected, so they can receive extra help.

Sometimes these suggestions help, but still students reach the practice environment without the language skills to succeed.

IPPEs and APPEs

In IPPE's, although we have to worry about patient safety, it's possible to catch language problems early enough to get help for students without slowing their progression through the pharmacy program. Unfortunately, however, given the grading and evaluation system in most IPPEs, a very low score on communication—which might make up 5% of the grade—will not give students a low enough grade overall to mandate remediation. In such cases, contact the college and explain that the student is a potential danger to patients and should be removed from the experience. This way, you can get help for the student so he can eventually succeed.

When students have a significant language deficit during advanced pharmacy practice experiences (APPEs), it's sadder because it means that throughout their years of pharmacy education, we've failed them. Lin, for example, made it through three years of pharmacy school without being able to communicate effectively with patients and other health care professionals. Even if his deficit isn't detected until late in his pharmacy education, we can't let him slide by with poor language skills. And even if we don't discover the problem until the end of his rotation with us, our obligation to patient care does not stop. If he graduates and enters practice, patients could be harmed or killed.

Possible Solutions

What can be done? Options are limited, and students with poor language skills need specialized help. Here's what you might do for Lin:

- Check with the university system, if your college of pharmacy is part of one. Most have an English language institute to help people whose speaking and comprehension are not up to par. Lin may require months of work to see results, and there are no guarantees, but at least he will get focused attention. He may need to take a leave of absence from the pharmacy program and pay extra for intensive language training.
- Help Lin recognize that the problem is real and must be addressed if he wants to be a practicing pharmacist. Emphasize real consequences, such as what happened, or could have happened, to a patient because of his language deficits.
- If you are the one who identified Lin's language deficits (typically by listening to complaints from patients and providers and observing patient care activities), stay involved. You don't have to commit significant time, but having someone from the practice environment check on him, meet with him regularly, and practice English with him in a real-world environment can help him stay focused on his goals.

Case 3

Student Lack of Focus

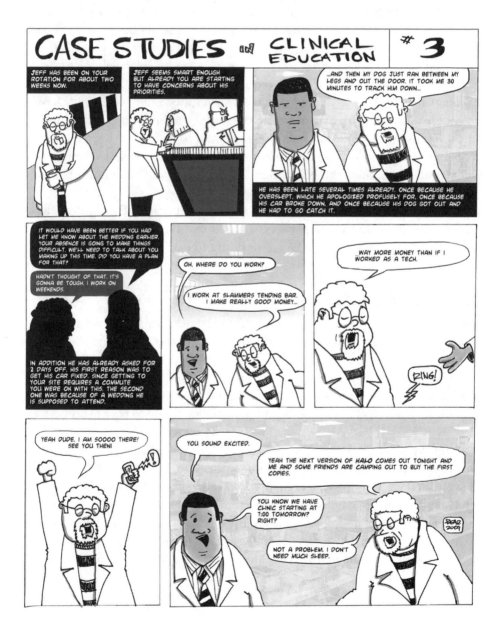

Here we see a student distracted by the world around him. He doesn't lack focus entirely—he's just not focused on the things we expect him to focus on.

Although of course there are exceptions, typical pharmacy students are around 21 to 23 years old when they start pharmacy school and enter introductory pharmacy practice experiences (IPPEs). They are 24 to 26 when they start advanced pharmacy practice experiences (APPEs). Students this age can be distracted by many things: relationships, entertainment, hobbies, work. Older students who come to pharmacy after other careers can have as many distractions, if not more, because they are likely to have family responsibilities.

Students may find themselves juggling responsibilities and desires. They have to choose between doing something necessary for their pharmacy education and something at home—or something they want to do for fun. Even if it is not a direct *this* versus *that* choice, it may be, as in Jeff's case, a choice between doing or not doing something that interferes with preparation or performance.

Jeff's decision to stay out late to pick up Halo with his pals will most likely lead to very little sleep and a poor showing the next day. He is betting on his ability to cope with his lack of sleep against his desire to play the new game.

Learning Experiences, Full-Time Work

As is evident in Jeff's situation, paid work may be necessary from a financial point of view, but it's also a huge distraction. An APPE is a full-time job itself. Having too much going on can lead to a series of excuses. Jeff may have been late to the pharmacy for the reasons he stated, but possibly other things are getting in the way of him doing what he should, such as choosing to stay out late with friends, trying to squeeze in too much, or failing to plan his time.

Certain skills necessary for success in a pharmacy experience are the same ones necessary for success in life. If your car needs maintenance but you keep putting it off to do things that are more fun, and your car breaks down, the problem is not the car, but your failure to carry out an important task at the right time. Young people accustomed to the flexibility of didactic coursework, with days that are rarely completely full, may not learn lessons about time and task management until confronted with their first full-time rotation.

Technology Steals Focus

I think some people would have phantom limb pain if they were separated from their mobile devices for more than a few minutes. Today, distracters are not left at home anymore, but instead come with students to the practice site via cell phones, smart phones, iPads, and iPods. These distractions infiltrate our lives.

Recently a friend introduced me to a little phone game where you can play Scrabble against each other. Seems fine, right? I like Scrabble. We started a game. The turns are slow and the next person may not get a chance to play for minutes or hours. I started a game with another friend. Still kinda slow. Then I found out you can start games with random individuals. Soon I had five games running and was constantly checking to see if anyone had played their next move.

Now, has Scrabble become a bad game? No. But normally it takes place for a finite amount of time and is over. Today, you can have your time and focus stolen from you in countless ways that were not available when many of us were in school—such as the Scrabble phone game as well as Twitter, Facebook, fantasy sports leagues, computer gaming, texting, and blogging.

Too Much of a Good Thing

Other distractions might include laudable activities such as serving as an officer in a student organization, participating in community service groups, being elected to student government, and taking part in committees. Such activities are likely to make the student a better pharmacist in the long run, unless they take up so much time that they become a barrier to actually becoming a pharmacist.

Years ago I had a student who was an amazing organizer and led so many group projects that she lost sight of the goal. She assumed that she would be able to keep up with her coursework, and she was wrong, ending up in academic jeopardy and eventually leaving the pharmacy program. I am sure that if she had become a pharmacist her leadership skills would have taken her far. But she could not give up short-term distractions in her journey to reach her long-term goal.

Probe the Situation

Working with unfocused students can be difficult because the root cause is not readily ascertainable. First, try to get a better handle on the diagnosis.

- Call the college, explain what you are seeing, and ask if anyone there has insight into the behavior that might help you.
- Ask the student about it. Results will vary, because some students will think that acknowledging their distraction is an admission of guilt, but you might try something like the approach below:

"Jeff, I wanted to talk to you because I am concerned that you don't seem to be giving this experience or my patients your full attention. Your focus seems to be elsewhere. When your mind is focused here and now on the patients, you do well, but sometimes you seem scattered. You've been late several times and occasionally seem distracted by things you would rather be doing. Is something going on in your life that would lead to this?"

Most likely Jeff will reiterate all the excuses about why he was late. You can say:

"Individually those are understandable reasons for being late, but they add up to a trend I am not happy with. They point to a lack of ability to spend adequate time preparing for each day. Is there something causing that?"

He might bring up outside factors causing problems, but the lack of focus may be nothing more than the distracters we talked about, which he is unlikely to admit. You might continue this way:

"Here is what I am asking you to do. For the rest of this experience, I want you to pay special attention to focusing on your duties here as a student. This includes being on time, being well rested, and being prepared for each day. With the ability that you have displayed so far when you are properly focused, I have no doubt that you will be successful if you do. If not, I am not so sure."

This is the starting point of the conversation. From here it's a good idea to remind Jeff of specific requirements of the experience so he clearly knows your expectations and the consequences of not meeting them. Be sure to document the encounter in writing and send a copy to the college's director of experiential education.

After having this talk, two things typically happen. The student will:

- See that what he is doing is not working and modify his behavior, either because he recognizes the need for improvement (intrinsic motivation) or doesn't want to risk the consequences (extrinsic motivation).
- Continue the same behavior pattern because he is too bound up in the distractions to untangle himself or does not believe that he will suffer the consequences.

Real vs. Possible Problems

What gets tricky is when the student alters his behavior appropriately, and after some time, has a *real* distraction that causes him to exhibit the same behavior again. Things happen. But now we're seeing the very behavior we said we would not stand for. So, what is our response?

Investigate. Ask for documentation that confirms the situation, such as doctor's note or plumber's receipt. If the corroboration is weak, you may need to impose the consequences fully and let him know that his history produced this result, not the single event. One lapse would not have been an issue without prior problems.

Some people are better at juggling life than others. They have an amazing ability to do many things at once and make the best use of time each day. Without evidence of detrimental effects, preceptors shouldn't jump the gun on cautioning students with many outside activities. How would you feel if you were accused of something that *might* happen rather than *did* happen? Wait for the problems to appear before attempting correction.

Case 4

Mismatched Expectations

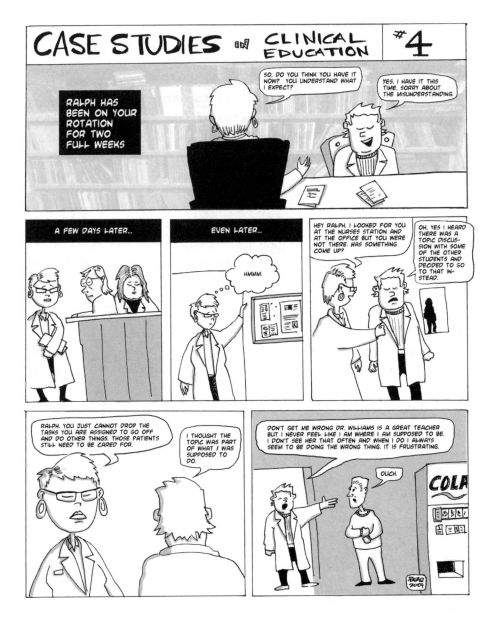

In Chapter 3 we talked about the importance of using the syllabus, calendar, orientation, and evaluation process to set and communicate expectations for students. In the scenario on page 97, Ralph and his preceptor are operating under different sets of expectations about Ralph's role in the experience, which is frustrating both of them.

Possible Causes

Where did this gap in perceptions come from?

- Ralph's past history may be a key factor. Like many pharmacy students, he has probably worked in or had education experiences in other pharmacies before. Regardless of practice area, every pharmacy has a system, culture, organizational style, and flow. He may have formed assumptions based on how he has seen things done before.

- Ralph may have talked informally with others—"rumor-mill research"—about what the norm is for this experience and has received misinformation based on a time when things were done differently. Maybe the rotation has evolved since then, or maybe it undergoes seasonal changes that Ralph didn't take into consideration during his research.

- If Ralph is not the only student at the site, the other students may be precepted by different faculty or may be at different points in their curriculum, and therefore what is true for them is not true for Ralph. Looking to these other students as a source of information about what he should be doing at any given time may result in guidance that is not wrong for them, but is wrong for Ralph.

- The root cause could be a primary misunderstanding of the words "may," "will," "can," and "should" in the assignment of the tasks. Ralph may have interpreted elective opportunities as mandatory, or vice versa.

The reason could also be a purposeful attempt to ignore the assigned tasks. If Ralph is uncomfortable enough with what he's supposed to do, he might occupy himself with other activities instead, thus avoiding discomfort while feeling that he is still participating. Then, when confronted, he can still

show that he was doing something, which feels better than shirking the work directly. This scenario sometimes happens when a student has previous work experience in a familiar setting.

For example, if you know that a student in a community pharmacy rotation has a great deal of experience as a technician, you might assign tasks that are less familiar, such as preparing educational information and providing detailed diabetic counseling. Even so, you may find him helping with the dispensing process at every opportunity. When you ask why, he proclaims how busy the pharmacy is and how much the tech staff needs help.

Is it possible the help was valuable? Yes. Did it allow him to avoid one task by doing a more familiar one? Also, yes.

When reminded of tasks they are supposed to be doing, students in this scenario will go back to them, but the pull of the familiar will always be there, which is why I prefer not to schedule students in locations where they have already had work experience. It is far too easy for both students and preceptors to forget the educational objectives because the students are so valuable in the role they played as employees.

Be Specific

One solution is to be very specific in your instructions. For our example, "I already know you can fill prescriptions, so I don't want you working on that unless I specifically ask you to. Spend your time on the tasks I assign you." Depending on just how uncomfortable the student is with the assigned task, you may need to say this more than once.

If the problem is lack of interest, refer to Case 1 for possible solutions.

Sometimes, the problem may be that the preceptor missed the boat on explaining complex work relationships at the site. For example, perhaps precepting is being carried out by a team, but only one name is listed as preceptor for the sake of convenience. The student may be unsure about whom he should take direction from and therefore may not understand priorities. When the "primary" preceptor gives the student a task, he may think that task has a higher priority, even if in reality it is optional or of significantly lower priority.

You can avoid or correct this situation by doing the following:

- Clearly detail who the student's supervisors are and which tasks or type of assignment each supervisor is responsible for.
- Provide a prioritized list of duties the student is supposed to perform.
- Stress how important it is for members of the precepting team to communicate with each other so that conflicting assignments are not given. If tasks are clearly outlined but one preceptor regularly interrupts with a new task to supersede the rest without consulting the other preceptors, frustration will worsen.

Autonomy, Perceptions

Sometimes expectations regarding level of autonomy can be part of the problem. In Chapter 7, I mentioned how student evaluations for one of my preceptors revealed that students disliked the level of autonomy he gave them. A student who has only been on highly structured rotations and goes to work with a preceptor who expects students to manage their own time may find the experience frustrating. The opposite can also be true.

Students' previous experiences will influence their expectations about your time. If they're used to being connected to the preceptor's hip because of space, duties, or convenience, they may view close oversight as normal. If things are looser at your site, students may feel that they don't see you enough, which feels bad to them—when in fact it's just different.

Maybe the students' work area at their first few rotations was very close to the preceptor, allowing for casual conversation during the day, while at your site it is located on another floor of the building and they only see you when specific interaction is necessary. They may feel that they lack a connection with you.

On the other hand, students used to distance who suddenly find themselves with you constantly may feel like you are looking over their shoulder all the time. They may chafe at the perceived lack of trust in them.

During orientation, bring up the level of oversight students can expect and ac-knowledge differences from what they have experienced before. This way, they will find the situation easier to accept even if they don't particularly like it.

Checking and Correcting Expectations

It seems that Dr. Williams, the preceptor in the case, already tried to correct expectations verbally—which is a reasonable first step. When attempting to clarify expectations with Ralph, simply repeating them is not particularly helpful, especially if he did not understand them in the first place. Instead, using your well-developed communication skills, ask Ralph to tell you what he thinks is expected of him. You could also have Ralph put in writing what he understands he is expected to do hourly, daily, or weekly. If it differs from what you actually expect, ask him where his impressions came from. Knowing the reasons for Ralph's misunderstanding will make it much easier to correct.

If questions and discussions about expectations don't work, you could try structured briefings used in tandem with calendars, to-do lists, check sheets, or other tools. Ask Ralph to give you a daily calendar of activities each morning for your approval, which ensures that you have written documentation of his responsibilities for the day and gives him a detailed plan. This could be done by email or in person.

If Ralph cannot get on the same page with you after you've tried different ways to confirm expectations, then it's reasonable to consider his performance deficient. You must provide the appropriate feedback to help him understand the nature of his deficiencies, document it with the college, and possibly refer him for remediation. Without efforts to correct this problem, Ralph's inability to grasp and carry out tasks in accordance with expectations will haunt him. Helping him now will help every person he ever works for or with.

Case 5

Inappropriate Behavior

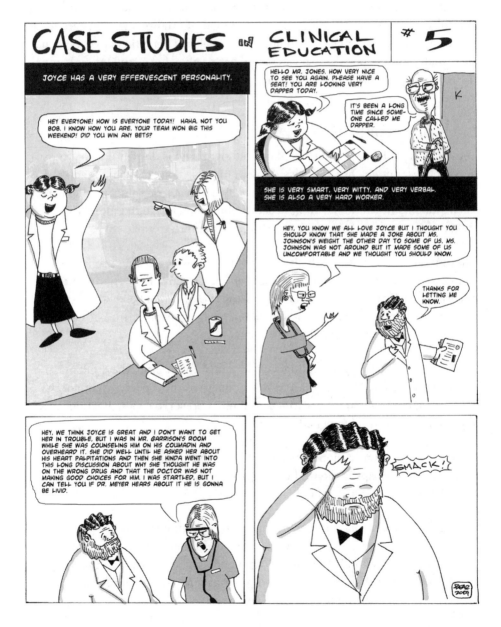

103

In this case, we talk about a variety of inappropriate behaviors. The most important point to take away is, never ignore any form of inappropriate behavior. Failing to correct problem behavior reinforces it—and the longer it continues, the greater the chance that patients or others will suffer ill effects from it.

Most inappropriate behaviors (with the exception of those similar to the scenario in the drawing on page 103) should be reported to both the college and the site's human resources (HR) department. Both organizations are likely to have procedures in place for handling these issues. Sanctions may be necessary, such as grade penalties, suspension, or not allowing a student back into the facility for education experiences.

Lack of Verbal Filters

Let's start with Joyce's situation. She's a student who is doing well from most perspectives, but she has some issues with impulse control. If you teach enough pharmacy students, you'll eventually come across someone like this. Such students mean no harm, but their inability to engage the filters that should exist between brain and mouth gets them into trouble.

They are not malicious and don't go out of their way to say inappropriate things to people; in fact, they may not even understand the inappropriateness of certain things they say. Rather than being their normal behavior, the tendency to say the wrong thing may happen when they are tired or nervous. They may realize their mistake after the fact.

To determine what we are dealing with, we must first talk to the student. In Joyce's case we have information from a concerned third party—a nurse that Joyce must continue to work with—so we must preserve goodwill while letting Joyce know what has happened.

Make the correction session as positive as possible. Start the conversation in a casual way, perhaps while walking together somewhere, or over lunch. It should go something like this:

> "Joyce, while we have a second, I wanted to mention something I think you can work on. As you know, we are a team here and everyone on the staff understands that we are trying to help you learn and improve. As such, I ask them regularly about your performance. I am happy to say that everyone really likes you and what you do here.

For the most part you are doing very well. The patients like you and the nurses and doctors seem very happy to have you around. We want this to continue. However, I got feedback from some of the staff that we need to discuss so you can continue to improve. I have two examples of things you've said off-handedly in conversation that could potentially get you in trouble, which we certainly don't want.

First, you were overheard making a joke about a patient the other day. You have a good sense of humor, which can help you build rapport with patients, but you must monitor yourself because, in our environment, you never know who is around. It could be very hurtful to patients or their families if they happened to overhear such a comment, and most likely you would never regain the relationship you had with them before.

Second, while you were talking to Mr. Garrison about his Coumadin, you gave the impression that his medication regimen was not right and his doctor was not providing the best care. I know that was probably not your intent, but this is the very point. We must be very careful about the impression we leave with our patients regarding the direction of their care. There is a trust relationship between patients and their health care providers we don't want to disrupt. Discussing differences of opinion or alternatives is something we should do together as a health care team before presenting options to the patient. Questioning the doctor's choices in front of Mr. Garrison could damage Mr. Garrison's trust in his doctor and also damage his doctor's ability to influence anything Mr. Garrison does regarding his health from here on out.

We very much want you to do well, and everyone here is looking out for your best interests. What I would like you to do is concentrate on slowing down a bit when you are communicating with others. Think about what you are about to say. I understand that silence can be uncomfortable, but little pauses to collect your thoughts are no problem and will give you a much better chance to phrase things in a way that avoids results you don't want. It is much better to say something right the first time than to have to apologize for it later. Can you do that for me?"

Such a conversation might devolve based on Joyce's acceptance of the facts. She might not agree with the assessment of inappropriateness, believing that what she did was innocent and not wrong. If so, you need to follow up by discussing perception and reality—something like:

> "Joyce, I understand that you don't see these events as a problem. That is your perception. Unfortunately, your perception isn't what matters in this case. It's the perception of the person you are communicating with that constitutes reality. As a health care professional, you must use your communication skills carefully to influence the perceptions of others. As it is, too few people exercise care when communicating with patients and members of the health care team. I need you to be one of those people."

Considering how Joyce has conducted herself so far, it's likely she would take the feedback well. However, she might express disappointment about colleagues giving you feedback without saying anything to her. It's not uncommon for students to feel betrayed when feedback comes from third parties who do not have direct responsibility for the evaluation. Emphasize that you would solicit this kind of feedback even if it had not been volunteered (in fact, the nurses in Joyce's situation had been instructed to provide feedback), and focus on improvement, not failure, to take out some of the sting.

Feedback won't necessarily work. It may be difficult for Joyce to change her ways if she has a habit of shooting from the hip verbally or her behavior is triggered when she's nervous. After you speak to her, go back and let the nurses know about it, and ask them to continue monitoring her when you are not around. If the behavior is repeated, determine if it's intentional or accidental.

If she unintentionally repeats the behavior, point out the instances to Joyce—reinforcing how important it is for her to rectify the problem. If the behavior is a habit, correcting it will take time. The best you can hope for is a decrease in the number of incidents during your rotation and continued improvement as she moves through the rest of her experiences, which will help her avoid potentially damaging situations in practice later. But if no one bothers to mention the problem to her, she'll never improve at all.

In rare cases, a person repeats problem behavior on purpose after having been given feedback about it. If that happens, you need to call the college, which may handle professionalism violations in various ways, including grade penalties, removal from the experience, mandated apologies, or sensitivity training.

Substance Abuse

Pharmacy students, like many other health care professionals, are at increased risk for abusing drugs because drugs are so accessible. However, substance abuse is not limited to what's behind the counter in pharmacies. Alcohol is a major concern, as are nonprescription and street drugs. Times change, and the drugs of choice for each generation and region change, but the fact that some student pharmacists abuse drugs does not change.

It's not always obvious when students are impaired. Some may appear to function fairly well. Even so, it is never appropriate for a health professional to practice in an impaired state. Students who are impaired or caught in the act of using drugs or alcohol on site must be removed from the site, and the college must be contacted so that appropriate follow-up can be initiated.

If a student is caught stealing drugs from a pharmacy, normal police procedures should be initiated. Having someone arrested with whom you've been working is not comfortable, but avoiding the issue and hoping it gets better doesn't work. The student poses a danger to patients, and for all you know, no matter what the student tells you, it's not his or her first offense. We would be derelict in our duty if we allowed the student to move to another rotation and continue to do the same thing.

Sometimes the first inkling of substance abuse might be performance problems and classic signs such as absenteeism, tardiness, behavioral changes, and trouble with cognition or attention span. In such cases, contact the college and discuss your suspicions. This is not something you can deal with on your own. Depending on the evidence, the school may want you to continue to monitor the situation or may have you bring the student in for an assessment.

Contacting the college is important because you don't know the student's history. Perhaps this problem has come up before. Like other health care professionals, student pharmacists are not excluded from practice or education automatically when they have substance abuse problems, and often they can take advantage of programs in place for rehabilitation.

When students have gone through one of these programs, they may already have a plan in place for counseling and monitoring. In Florida, where I work, the Professionals Resource Network (PRN) runs the Impaired Practititioners Program, which collaborates closely with the board of pharmacy and colleges to help students with substance abuse problems. It assesses students and puts them in a monitored plan toward recovery, which can salvage their education and their pharmacy career. Your state may have a similar program.

Other Impairment

Impairment is anything that prevents students from operating at their normal level of cognition, whether short term or long term—such as someone suffering from a concussion or struggling with depression. Memory lapses and loss of problem-solving ability can be dangerous in a health care professional.

It is not your job to diagnose students with such problems or implement solutions. Your role is simply to identify behaviors or deficits that indicate a potential problem and to contact the college, which will investigate further, assess the student, and launch an action plan to help him or her.

In Florida, the same organization that monitors professionals with substance abuse issues, PRN, monitors people with other impairments. It defines "impairment" not only as use of or dependence on drugs or alcohol, but also "distorted thought processes resulting from mental illness or physical condition, or disruptive social tendencies."

Harassment

Harassment falls into two categories. Nonsexual harassment includes threats made against another person as well as persistent, unwelcome, or inappropriate contact with a colleague, patient, or others. Examples include a student who:

- Calls a physician at home to argue about a decision.
- Posts derogatory comments about a fellow student on his social networking page.
- Sends threatening statements to a colleague.

Such behaviors could point to an underlying problem or could be a giant misunderstanding, but the preceptor is not expected to sort things out. Simply identify the behavior and notify the college, which will follow the appropriate policies, and if a larger problem is detected, implement a plan.

For sexual harassment, every college will have a procedure in place, whether the student is the accused or the victim. Regardless of the circumstances, the preceptor's cooperation is required. Once the situation is reported, it's often out of the college's hands and taken over by an organization that investigates such events independently, to avoid bias.

For both types of harassment, I've found these significant challenges:

- **Getting the event reported.** People are often reluctant to report sexual harassment, and they feel vulnerable after coming forward. In experiential education, victims often believe the process is too bothersome, considering the short-term nature of the experience, to make an official complaint. I've noticed that when victims come forward, it's usually because they feel a civic responsibility to protect others. Once the college receives a report of an event, there is no turning back; it is obligated to follow up to the fullest extent of the process—but this should never stop us from reporting. If anything, the short duration of educational experiences should further our obligation, because serial harassers can hide their activities for a long time in such settings. For example, a student could take liberties with people at one site, then another, and then another—and if no one reports the behavior, not only are more victims exposed, but the student is never forced to recognize the inappropriateness of his or her behavior.

- **Understanding a site's social dynamics.** Let's face it, a close-knit community of colleagues often develops its own behavioral rules and limitations, regardless of what the HR department defines as appropriate. If students try to participate in conversations the way an insider would, they don't know where the boundaries lie and are unaware of potential pitfalls. For example, one student on rotation at a small hospital in a small town found himself working with a chatty group of nurses who'd been together a long time. They routinely made off-color comments and gossiped about friends and colleagues. After several weeks in this environment he felt comfortable enough to participate—and he was charged with sexual harassment. Joining their bawdy conversation was a poor choice, and I am not excusing such behavior, but the student could have avoided trouble if his preceptor had warned him about the dynamic in the first place.

Failure to Maintain Patient Confidentiality

Students are bombarded by training related to the Health Insurance Portability and Accountability Act (HIPAA) from their first entry into pharmacy school. Despite the training and constant reminders about HIPAA policies and patient confidentiality, students still violate HIPAA. Colleges and rotation sites have well-documented procedures for handling HIPAA violations, which must be followed to the letter to reduce the consequences to both victims and students. When violations occur, the privacy offices at the college and the site will want to investigate, and they may impose sanctions.

Improper Dress and Appearance

The syllabus and accompanying documentation for the experience should clearly detail what constitutes appropriate dress and accessories, including clothing, hair, jewelry, tattoos, and piercings. When a student repeatedly violates the dress code, you need to intervene. If you feel uncomfortable because the student is of the opposite sex, consider bringing in a same-sex colleague to talk with the student.

Making the conversation about patient care and being a successful practitioner steers it away from your personal opinion. When I hold these conversations, I point out that a student pharmacist's dress should not be so distracting that it prevents people from absorbing things they need to know. Patients and health care providers will not get necessary information if they are too busy looking at what students are wearing to listen to them. In short, appearance should not have a negative effect on patient care.

The student's perception of what is "distracting" is not at issue; it is the person *being distracted* that matters. Some people seem to be unaware of what is distracting and inappropriate to others and have trouble policing themselves. Such students need pointed directions about maintaining an appropriate appearance in your setting. If they fail to uphold those standards, send them home and contact the college. You have a responsibility to protect your practice and cannot afford to have a student's dress reflect poorly on your service.

Excessive Texting and Phone Calls

In today's world, students expect to be connected electronically at all times. Texting, talking to friends on the phone, and accessing social networking sites are constant sources of temptation—which may distract students from their duties and cause them to miss deadlines.

Outline policies regarding texting and personal calls at the beginning of the experience. Quickly deal with minor violations, such as too many breaks to answer calls or respond to friends, so they don't continue or escalate. Egregious violations, which include texting while on rounds or taking a call during a counseling session, require a focused intervention in which you discuss the behavior and consequences and ask the student to apologize to the people affected, including patients and colleagues. Students who allow themselves to be distracted by technology may lack engagement in the experience, similar to Maya in Case 1, and may need to be dealt with accordingly.

Of course, texts and cell phone calls themselves are not bad—it's how they are used. We don't want to leave the impression with students that using technology in the clinical setting is not valuable, but it needs to be channeled so it adds to our ability to care for patients rather than competing for our time.

Case 6

When Bad Things Happen to Good People

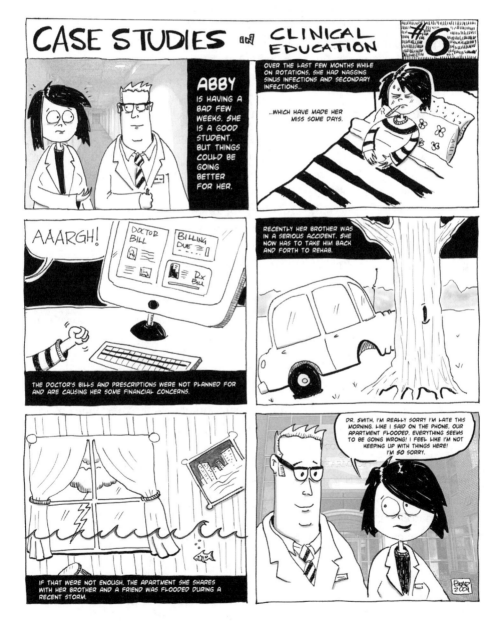

People lead complex lives, in or out of pharmacy school. Even though the scenario in the illustration may seem exaggerated, I've seen cases this bad—and worse.

Students going through significant life events, like Abby is, can exhibit the same symptoms as someone who is unmotivated or unfocused—but the cause is entirely different. For preceptors, recognizing the difference between excuses and legitimate reasons can be very hard. We want to believe that our students are telling us the truth about their trials and tribulations. We have to tread a line between asking for proof and being sympathetic.

Documentation and Continuity

The best approach is straightforward; ask for documentation such as a doctor's note, an accident report, and a picture of the flooding. These are easy enough for the student to acquire and should not be a burden. You might feel uncomfortable requesting such things, not wanting to imply deceit and insult the student. It's easier if you make providing documentation a standard approach when students are absent. Students will be fine with it, and it's worse if you *don't* ask for documentation and discover one of them lying to you. If that happens, the uncomfortable feeling will be your constant wondering if *any* of them are telling the truth, which, in my opinion, is much worse.

If you're really having a hard time asking for documentation, throw the college under the bus. Tell students that the college is always after you about documentation (and we are).

Once you confirm that the problem is real, think about its effect on the quality of the student's experience. How much disruption can your experience absorb and still maintain its integrity? It's up to you to decide.

One key factor in your decision will be how important continuity is to the educational quality of the experience. Some rotations are set up so that continuity is not a big deal. Whether something happens today or tomorrow doesn't matter, as long as it gets done. In other rotations, interruptions in continuity of care can really undermine educational objectives.

Making Up Missed Time

If your experience can survive lapses in continuity, then how will missed opportunities be made up? The question is not *if* they will be made up, but *when*. In most cases, options for makeup work are limited. The most common options are:

- **Nights or longer days.** Frankly, I have trouble stomaching this as a choice. Here is why. Students should be using this time to prepare for the next day. Allowing them to apply these hours toward makeup experience means that they are missing out on preparation time. Not the best option, in my opinion.

- **Weekends and holidays.** This option doesn't intrude into the time that students would typically be spending at the rotation site. But it's not a good course of action if the student is expected to make up activities that don't happen on weekends or holidays, or if you have certain supervision goals for the student and you won't be there during those times. If, however, the site's needs and processes on weekends and holidays are similar to what the student missed, and someone you trust to supervise him or her will be present, it should work out fine. Just remember that a student with difficulties like the ones in this case may need the weekend to work through them.

- **Gaps between experiences.** All students have breaks in their rotation schedules. For introductory experiences, breaks might be at the end of a semester, and for advanced experiences, they might be during scheduled time off throughout the year, although breaks vary for each college. Each student's schedule differs, as well. The viability of having students make up time during a break depends on how far away the break is from the experience and how much the loss in continuity will affect the educational objectives. For example, if Abby's next scheduled break is seven months from now, she'll need time to get back up to speed. Making up the time on a 1 to 1 ratio is hard to justify and the preceptor may need to alter the ratio to accommodate the loss of continuity, adding an extra day or two for time to relearn the workflow. If the days she missed are being replaced with days spent simply relearning the system, it's not an adequate replacement.

- **Makeup projects.** The big benefit of assigning makeup projects is that students can complete them over time while on other rotations. It's a workable solution in the face of scheduling concerns, but has problems of its own. Such projects should have rigor. They require significant attention from students, which means students must divert attention from their current experience—not a good thing for someone who already has time issues caused by outside problems. They may *want* to do it this way and feel very strongly that they can, but is adding another task to an already full plate a good idea?

Whatever makeup method you choose, give students the same attention as if the experience hadn't been disrupted. This means supervision, deadlines, feedback, and evaluation. When one student leaves an experience, it's easy to put most of our attention on the next student, even if the previous student needs to make up time or activities.

If we are not careful, the makeup path becomes an easier path. Should that become known, students could be tempted to vie for that path, too. To avoid this, be sure that makeup work is at least as rigorous as the original task.

Halting the Experience

A point arrives when it's not possible to make up the experience. If you think you are close to this point, check with the college. Colleges typically have strict limits on how much can be lost before the experience needs to be stopped and restarted later. Such policies help you know the critical point at which to intervene.

If you can't salvage the experience, it's time to hit the reset button. It sounds harsh, but it's actually the compassionate thing to do. Students in Abby's situation may have a locus of control skewed highly to the internal side (see Chapter 9). They believe they are in control of everything, and if they push a little more, try a little harder, they can make it work out. But sometimes pushing more and trying harder just makes things worse. Students in these situations sometimes need someone to step in and protect them from themselves.

Is this a paternalistic viewpoint? Maybe, but I ask you, if you found someone banging his head on a wall, would you assume he's trying to tear it down and help him out by pushing the back of his head? Or would you try to get him to stop?

Students may not realize how close they are to a meltdown. Time away from an experience to fix their problems and get back on track can make a huge difference to their health and future performance. Key points to make when talking with the student include:

- You have missed too much of this experience to make it up.
- You have too much going on in your life at the moment to be successful in this experience.
- We need to reschedule you for another time while you use this time to take care of your problems.
- If you don't take this time, you are never going to get on top of the situation and your next rotation will just end up like this one.

Of course, if a student is having issues like Abby's but is getting along without missing significant time and activities, we can only counsel her about the possibility of taking a break.

When Health Is at Stake

Intervening to help students is especially important when their health is in question. In my typically melodramatic mode, I tell students, "To become a licensed pharmacist, you first have to be a *live* pharmacist. They don't give licenses to dead people." Students with health concerns may be able to survive one or two experiences only to become more ill and then crash, thus missing even more time than if they'd tended to their health earlier. In addition, health problems affect performance and performance affects patient care.

Think about a student on an advanced pharmacy practice experience (APPE) who gets mono. His doctor recommends several weeks of rest, but the student doesn't want to graduate late and ignores the advice. He participates in his APPE anyway. His recuperation time stretches from weeks to months. His energy level is very low, and the stress of not doing as well as he would like mounts up. He continues on his scheduled APPEs but eventually doesn't pass an APPE because he can't keep up with the work. Now he's still sick, but must also make up the APPE he failed. If he'd been counseled to step away for the recommended rest, this might have been avoided.

These situations happen all the time. I see several each year. Students have the same likelihood of developing long-term debilitating illnesses as anyone else in their demographic—and maybe more, if you consider the effect stress has on the potential for illness. Accidents are prevalent among this age group, too.

If it's decided that a student will leave an experience to sort things out or get healthy again, your job as a preceptor is done. With one caveat. No matter how long they were with you and what type of relationship you developed with them, it makes a difference when such students hear the following from you:

- You wish them well in their endeavors to "right the ship."
- Once they get everything settled, you would be happy to have them back.

It is the sentiment that is helpful, not the outcome. Maybe you will never see the student again. Logistically, coming back to repeat the experience with you may not be possible. But letting the student know that leaving the experience does not equate to failure on his or her part can make a huge difference. Don't underestimate the value of a few kind words.

Case 7

Academic Dishonesty

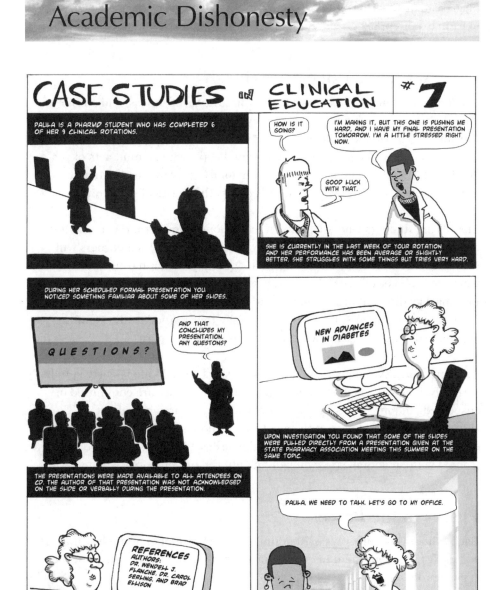

Academic dishonesty has to do with a student gaining unfair advantage over other students, resulting in an inaccurate assessment of his or her actual level of skills, abilities, or knowledge. Most of the time, academic dishonesty involves plagiarism or cheating on tests or quizzes, but forms of academic dishonesty exist in experiential education that may not be quite so common elsewhere.

Take Academic Honesty Seriously

Academic dishonesty indicates a lack of maturity, selfishness, and possibly a flawed character. It shows that the person is willing to break the rules to get the outcome he or she wants and reflects a lack of integrity that does not jibe with the tenets of the pharmacy profession. People who commit acts of academic dishonesty are demonstrating an inability to overcome the temptation of taking an easy path rather than the *right* path in critical situations.

Identifying students who are guilty of infractions is important, because if they cheat in their academics, what will they do in practice? What corners will they cut? What will they do to save time or money? What harm will come from these choices? Recently, cases have been reported in the news in which pharmacists diverted drugs, substituted active ingredients, or diluted drugs to increase their profits. I think it's fair to say that a student who commits academic dishonesty is already taking steps down this path.

As clinical faculty members, preceptors must take academic honesty standards seriously, follow through when acts of academic honesty are committed or suspected, and make sure the proper consequences are carried out. To do this, you need to understand the academic dishonesty policies of the student's college or university. Start by learning the basics and then, if you ever are confronted with an actual case, you can find out the full processes and protocols.

Phases in the Process

Each school's specific ways of handling academic dishonesty will be different, so I can't talk about them in detail, but below is an outline of phases in the typical process.

- **Identification**. This is the point where the preceptor identifies a problem. "Something is rotten in the state of Denmark," as it were.

Sometimes you might need to talk with the college to determine whether the event in question is truly academic dishonesty, but more than likely if you have to ask, it is.

- **Investigation**. In this phase, information and documentation are compiled, including gathering evidence from witnesses. Depending on the school, the approach may vary. You may need to gather your evidence so you can present the case, but the school may require a third party to investigate and review the evidence, as well.

- **Charging**. Once the investigation is completed and the evidence is considered strong enough to pursue, the student must be informed that he or she is being charged with academic dishonesty. The student is presented with the evidence and informed of the process that will follow.

- **Adjudication**. The student is presented with the possible consequences and given the opportunity to accept the outcome, defend himself or herself, question the evidence, and so on. Unlike a criminal law situation, in which governing laws and processes are in place, each university will have its own specific process to follow—ranging from a form filled out and signed by student and faculty documenting the event, to a full-blown academic honor court. A prior history of academic dishonesty may bring the student stiffer penalties. Some schools have zero tolerance or a strict "one and done" policy.

- **Penalty**. The penalty associated with an event will be decided during the adjudication phase and then implemented—a process that may or may not involve you. If the penalty is the loss of points or letter grades, you would take care of it, but the college or university would handle penalties such as failing a course, suspension, or expulsion.

The phases described above may involve a long, drawn-out process or they may be rolled together. At our university, if significant evidence suggests that a student with no prior history committed an act of academic dishonesty, the student is presented with a form stating the event, the evidence of his or her guilt, and the penalty to be imposed. If the student accepts the outcome, he or she signs the form and the penalty is implemented. Or the student can ask for a hearing, which triggers the complete process, with all phases.

The Experiential Setting

The scenario above involves a situation in which Paula used slides verbatim from another person's slide show, without any acknowledgement. She appears to be guilty of plagiarism, which can occur in presentations, papers, or any project that is supposed to be original and created by the student. Because projects, papers, and presentations are common in experiential education, I've found that plagiarism is one of the most typical types of academic dishonesty during rotations. Frankly, I believe this to be mostly due to ignorance rather than deceitful intent. We educators need to do a better job of instructing our students about plagiarism, starting in high school.

Paula's academic dishonesty may have been intentional or through ignorance, but either way, some form of intervention needs to be made. The preceptor in this case has already done some investigating. She probably needs to ask Paula for a complete reference list from her presentation to see if Paula left some off accidentally, in which case, a milder penalty is in order. Even so, she needs to follow the steps for reporting academic dishonesty.

The preceptor should contact the school to find out if Paula had prior academic dishonesty incidents. Let's assume she did not. The preceptor should compile the evidence from her investigation and think about penalties appropriate for the case, with guidance from the school. Then she should sit down with Paula, preferably with a third party as a witness, and present her evidence and assessment of why the references were missing, along with an explanation of the penalty. (Typical options would be a zero for the presentation; lowering the rotation grade; failing the APPE; writing a paper on academic dishonesty, plagiarism, or ethics; or giving written or verbal apologies to the audience or original authors.) Paula could either accept the outcome of the preceptor's findings or ask for a formal hearing.

Cheating on quizzes or tests can also occur in experiential education, but you usually don't have to worry too much about students getting answers from each other during quizzes and tests because so few students are taking them—it's easy to seat them far apart. However, if you use a standard test and rarely change it, students might get hold of the test's content in advance.

In experiential settings, subtle forms of academic dishonesty involve ways that students gain "unfair advantage" leading to inaccurate assessment of their knowledge and skills. For example, it's academic dishonesty if students:

- Say they were at their rotation site until a certain time, as directed, but in reality, they left early, which means they did not comply fully with performance expectations.
- Claim to have interviewed and provided education to X number of patients, but really only worked with half that number—so they're trying to get credit for something they didn't do.
- Are given an assignment to create an original presentation, oral or written, on a topic of their choice, but instead deliver the same presentation they did last month, without changes—failing to do original work.
- Violate a policy, such as the Health Insurance Portability and Accountability Act, and then lie to try to cover it up and avoid the consequences of their lapse.
- Call in sick when they are not, thus setting themselves up for a makeup experience that may be easier than the original work.

You may think that some of these examples stretch the definition a bit. However, experiential environments are very different from the educational setting where academic dishonesty guidelines were originally developed, so the guidelines must be adapted.

Preceptors must view each assignment and evaluation as a possible source of academic dishonesty, think how dishonesty would manifest itself in those contexts, and then, if we detect dishonesty, we must act. To do otherwise is to effectively ignore the situation. Ignoring it gives students the opportunity and temptation to bypass learning opportunities, producing students without the skills or knowledge they need. We must hold the line if we want to maintain educational integrity.

Academic dishonesty cases are uncomfortable, and it's tempting to try to avoid them or deal with them in-house, but you really need to document them and report them to the college because you don't have the student's full history.

First of all, he or she may be a serial cheater with several previous incidents on file—or a serial cheater whose wrongdoings have never been reported or documented. If you fail to report the incident, you have just added yourself to a long list of other faculty who probably did the same and allowed that student to continue his or her dishonest ways. For students like this to learn the consequences, their behavior must be reported.

Second, documenting such incidents through official channels protects you. For example, if you handled an instance of academic dishonesty by lowering the student's grade but did not report the situation to the college, a gap will exist between the evidence and the outcome if the student later disputes the grade. This could cause you more problems than documenting it correctly to begin with.

Third, even if it is the student's first offense, going through the proper process will instill in her an awareness of the event's seriousness and of your attitude regarding the behavior. Why does this matter? Those of us who are full-time faculty like to think we have some pull, but students hear us lecture them about academic honesty all the time. As a practicing pharmacist, you have a very different place in their minds. You are the real world. If you say academic honesty is important, they believe you more.

Fourth, reporting the incident, even if it's the student's first, establishes a history. It may give the student incentives to never be involved in another case. And if he or she does commit another offense, the college has grounds for more severe penalties.

Accidental Violations

As noted earlier, it's possible that Paula's academic dishonesty was accidental. I don't want to soften the line we have drawn, but mistakes happen.

Sometimes a student may be an innocent participant. For example, think of a situation in which student A is tutoring student B and discovers that student B turned in some work as her own that student A had created. It might look to the instructor as if student A were a part of the scheme. The truth should come out in the investigation phase, although it might not, which means that both people might end up going through the academic dishonesty process.

The college can help you with the investigation or even relieve you of the burden altogether, depending on the process it follows. Determining whether it was accidental or intentional is part of the academic dishonesty process and in the final analysis, even students who turn out to be innocent participants can learn a valuable lesson by going through the process's phases.

Case 8

Overconfident Students

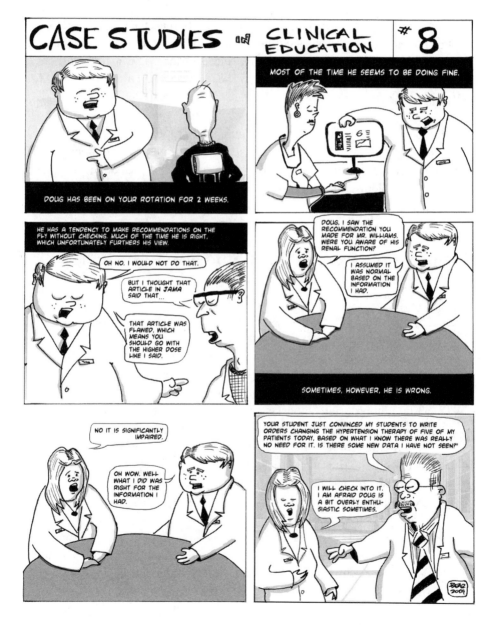

If you have ever had to deal with someone like Doug, you can imagine that such students create one of the most difficult situations for preceptors. Students with an inflated view of their abilities can be hard to identify, because they may be reasonably competent. Sometimes, you won't be able to tell if they are overconfident until something bad happens or a few events unfold that bring the problem to your attention.

Students who have confidence without the ability to match can be dangerous. People who come across as very confident can often convince someone, just because of their attitude of certainty, that they are right. This leads to others taking their recommendations even when they are wrong, which could lead to patient harm or death.

Compounding the issue is that such students have trouble seeing their own deficits and tend to put the blame elsewhere. If their self-confidence is extremely overblown, they may not only be in complete denial about the part they play in problems, but may also be convinced that people are conspiring to make them look bad.

Hallmarks of Overconfident Students

Some of the hallmarks of overconfident students are:

- Giving firm, yet wrong, answers to questions they are asked in education sessions, on the phone, on rounds, etc.
- Tending to want to be autonomous, whether it's part of the experience or not. For example, they may provide recommendations or educational information to patients or other health care providers without appropriate supervision, or make exceptions to defined policies without having the proper authority.
- Convincing others to believe the student's way is correct, when it isn't. We hope that health care providers would not be convinced to choose an incorrect course based on a student's autonomous recommendations, but if they are, it's another indicator of the student's confidence and persuasion skills.
- Giving multiple excuses for why things turned out differently than they expected and not believing that the discrepancy has anything to do with something *they* did wrong. In their minds, the only option is that an outside factor caused things to work out poorly.

- Blaming others when things do not go quite right, especially when they can't find adequate excuses to explain the error. The bigger the problem, the more blame there will be to spread around.
- Rarely, if ever, saying "I don't know," yet being wrong regularly. Student pharmacists should make steady progress toward knowing a significant number of answers, but it's a hyperbolic curve that will never reach maximum. Even experienced practicing pharmacists face questions they can't answer. When a student purports to know everything, it's a huge red flag.

Narrowing Down the Problem

When you work with students like this, gathering evidence from patient charts and conversations with other staff will be critical. You must show these students the consequences of their actions. Once you have detailed documentation, you should be able to narrow down the problem and understand its true source, which may be any of the issues below, or a combination.

- Is it a problem with the underlying knowledge base? Is the student unaware of having global knowledge deficiencies? Perhaps the real problem is being underprepared and not realizing it.
- Is it accelerated confidence? Maybe their knowledge base is pretty good, and they know it, but they fail to recognize that they still have more to learn.
- Is it an inability to admit their own limitations? Maybe they realize they have knowledge deficits, but act as if they know what they are talking about because they hate being perceived as inadequate.

Failure to Recognize Knowledge Deficits

Perhaps Doug excelled in his didactic studies, but now he is struggling to put it together clinically. Chapter 9 talked about how student pharmacists tend to encounter very few situations where they do poorly; no wonder they have confidence in their abilities. They may do fine in their first few advanced pharmacy practice experiences (APPEs), perhaps because the experiences are not overly complex, or they involve specific duties and information learned onsite as opposed to relying on their base knowledge. Then, when such students get to APPEs where their knowledge base is inadequate, they don't see it because they've done well so far.

Doug needs help recognizing his deficits. He needs to learn that he can fail and that there is a path to improvement. You must provide Doug with the opportunity to fail safely. Safety must remain top priority. If you have documented evidence of Doug giving wrong information, you could suspend his patient care activities—which will certainly get his attention. Then you can put him in a structured program to help him see his deficits. If his knowledge base as a whole is deficient, this should not be too hard. There are several ways to do this without endangering patients.

- Create a test covering areas in which his knowledge and skills are weak. Ask for specific answers that are not subject to interpretation. If his knowledge base is poor, he will not do well, which gives you the basis for a conversation about the potential negative outcomes that could result.

- Use real or fabricated case studies. Pull data from charts and have Doug work up cases. Again, if his knowledge base is poor, he'll have difficulty, opening the door to discuss the potential outcomes of his recommendations.

After Doug has failed several times in carefully controlled situations and agreed that he has deficits, you can slowly move him back into patient care areas, with very specific restrictions. For example: "Never write a note or talk to a person regarding patient care without me there." This could evolve into: "Never write a note or talk to a person regarding patient care without talking to me about it first." The goal is to get him back into the experience's normal way of operating.

Excessive Confidence

Students in this category know what they are doing for the most part, but may be so gung-ho about the profession and doing well that they overstep their bounds and end up in trouble. They may also have some specific deficits they don't recognize. You are likely to encounter such students later in their APPE cycle, and they probably have done very well along the way, which adds to their feeling of confidence and may prompt them to take risks, assuming they will be right.

Overconfident students can go through entire rotations without running into something they don't know, which is when their problem becomes evident.

And sometimes it's not that they are wrong, but unenlightened. Pharmacy faculty try hard to teach students that patient care should be based on the best possible evidence—known as evidence-based pharmacy. It's a good concept, but can work against students in some situations, such as Doug's. He meant to do good, but was overzealous—trying to convince others to change the way they do things based on evidence. But do they have all the evidence? Does his recommendation based on evidence he believes to be complete take into consideration the climate where those recommendations will be implemented, as well as specific variables of the site? Experienced practitioners know what to take into account when making decisions, whereas students may not. Students may believe they have it all down when in reality, they don't, which, unfortunately leads to conversations like that shown in the last panel of the case.

Removing such students from the practice environment may not be necessary. Your decision depends on the incidents that have happened so far and your personal judgment about lessons the student has learned from those experiences. You will need to make these students aware of the possibility of failure, but it's more difficult than with students unaware of their knowledge deficits, because a simple test or case study exercise will not allow them to see the problem.

Dive into specific deficits to expose them to the student. Pick out cases where the *right* choice may not be *right*, and where the *evidence* does not match the *best choice.* Students are likely to find this painful. They will not be happy with the process and may question whether you are right. The road to the poor outcome may be much harder to see, and thus much harder to show them, but it's the only way to help them understand the distance they still must go to grasp the intricacies of practice.

In the last panel of the case study above, Doug convinced a physician's medical students to change orders for patients with hypertension—perhaps bringing them closer to the recommended guidelines for hypertension therapy. Let's assume that no overt problem existed with the current therapy. Imagine this scenario:

> The physician in question is Doctor Zhivago, head of cardiology for the hospital and chair of the Pharmacy & Therapeutics Committee. He has been mildly resistant to including pharmacists in making decisions for his patients, but has softened over time after seeing some helpful interactions and improvements in care. Politically, pharmacy needs to continue

building his support. It's true that the hypertension therapy
for his five patients could have been improved slightly on
paper, but the current therapy was working and Dr. Zhivago's
attitude toward pharmacy interventions had improved. Now,
Doug's changes could dampen Dr. Zhivago's goodwill and
hamper the inclusion of pharmacy in future decision-making,
which could limit pharmacists' ability to prevent or solve
much larger problems.

Of course, if those five patients were in real jeopardy, making changes would
have been the right thing to do, but in this situation, after all the variables
are weighed, the better choice is to maintain the current therapy. Pharmacy
is not practiced in a vacuum, and sometimes preceptors isolate students from
issues related to the site's interpersonal and political landscape. But if students
understand the dynamics of the environment in which they are practicing,
they can see the potential pitfalls of failing to consider these dynamics when
making decisions.

Inability to Admit Limitations

Although it hasn't happened often, I've encountered a few students who need
to believe they are right at all costs. They are difficult to deal with—and even
dangerous. I'm no psychologist, as I said earlier in this book, but I wonder if
students who exhibit this behavior have an underlying psychological problem
that has gone unidentified.

Students who display this behavior will do the same things as other students
with confidence problems—making errors and being confident that they were
doing the right thing. The difference is that if you provide them with evidence,
they will make excuses or divert the blame instead of accepting that it was
their fault. When multiple sources of evidence are shown, they will argue that
the situation was unfair to them and they are being singled out for persecution.
When they have a success they will immediately point out that they are right
as proof of the rightness of their view.

With this kind of student, the resolution is rarely easy and may take the
concerted effort of multiple preceptors and the college. At first, the situation
should be handled as for the other types of overconfident students described
earlier. For all you know, the student is one of those types. Only after you
have presented evidence of the student's failures and he or she doesn't accept

them will you find out that you are dealing with a different and much more difficult situation.

You can follow the same steps as with Doug in the section "Failure to Recognize Knowledge Deficits" and suspend such students from participating in clinical practice. More than likely, however, they will not see their suspension as a result of their poor performance and inability to improve, but instead, as unjust punishment.

Students like this use any excuse possible to explain why they are not responsible. They blame others. They may try to gain support from others to show how well they are doing. They may even lie about things they did or did not do to cover their failures.

Occasionally, they will accede to some point of error, but only to lend strength to their other denials. Personally, I think these are all stalling tactics in an effort to delay remediation. They know they have a limited time with you and hope to squeak through and move on their next rotation.

Techniques discussed above for helping students recognize where they need to improve won't work for students in this category. Give them a test or case study, and if they do poorly they'll deem it unfair. Show them that their decisions led to poor outcomes, and they'll find others to blame or deny that the outcome was their fault.

If you find yourself with a student like this, contact the college as soon as you can. This student's performance needs a hard look across all APPEs and coursework; maybe he or she has exhibited similar issues all along but managed to get by. Based on the college's broad view of the student's performance, initiating remediation may be possible.

Probably the best thing that could happen to such students is stopping their progress in pharmacy school and referring them for mental health counseling. I don't say that lightly. Until they come to terms with the possibility that they could do great harm by failing to admit mistakes, they will never be successful pharmacists. They will continue to be a danger to their patients, their practice, and their employer.

Now that I've planted a picture in your mind of this sort of problem, try not to see it in every student when it's not really there. In 20 years, I've run into it only a few times. *Healthy* confidence is a good thing. We want students to build confidence over time, so that when they step into the wide world of pharmacy they know when to trust their knowledge and skills and when to seek more information. Although students with *a bit* too much confidence can be a problem, we have the opportunity to teach them how to temper their confidence and progress toward their goal of being successful pharmacists.

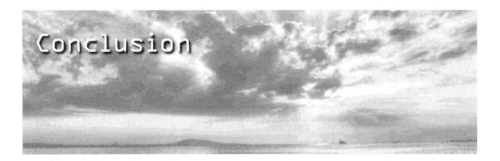

Conclusion

Well, this is the end of the book. I hope you've gotten something useful out of it. Before you put it down, I'd like to mention a few more things.

Final Tips

1. **Pick this book back up again.** It is designed to be used when you need help, not just to be read through once and tossed. Maybe some points I've made don't really apply to you now, but they might in the future. So keep this book handy.

2. **Feel free to disagree.** As I told you in the preface, this book stems from a series of conversations I've held with preceptors over the years. Although I have experience, I don't have every answer. Alternative viewpoints are possible. If something suggested in this book doesn't work for you, explore other options.

3. **Never forget your priorities.** Patient, Student, Profession. If you remember these, you have a great chance of being a good preceptor. But don't just remember the order, because although patients come first, all three priorities are intertwined. Pharmacists who take care of their patients also protect their profession and provide opportunity for their students. Pharmacists who protect their profession protect patients and students in the long term. Pharmacists who protect students help students become what they should be, and in doing so protect their patients and their profession.

4. **Stay in touch with the college or colleges that supplies students for your rotations.** Not just when things are going bad or you need something. Drop a line when things are going well, when new things are happening, and when some milestone has been reached. Honestly, we love to hear good things, too. It makes the day much brighter.

5. **Stay in touch with other preceptors.** Form groups either through the college or on your own that allow you to share ideas and support each other. It's easier to improve when you don't have to think of everything yourself. Isolating yourself means you are responsible for every improvement—an undue burden you shouldn't put on yourself.

6. **Stay in touch with your students.** You want to feel fulfilled? Keep tabs on them as they grow in the profession. Every patient they help, you helped, too.

Helpful Resources

Reading this book will not necessarily make you a better preceptor, but it might, if you try out its ideas. Below are listed other books that provide a different view or more detail.

Good luck in your adventures in precepting!

Books for Preceptors

- Cuéllar LM, Ginsburg DB, eds. *Preceptor's Handbook for Pharmacists.* 2nd ed. Bethesda, Md: American Society of Health-System Pharmacists; 2009.

- Alguire PC, DeWitt DE, Pinsky LE, et al., eds. *Teaching in Your Office: A Guide to Instructing Medical Students and Residents.* 2nd ed. Philadelphia: American College of Physicians Press; 2008.

Books Providing Insight into Students

- Stein SM, ed. *Boh's Pharmacy Practice Manual: A Guide to the Clinical Experience.* 3rd ed. Philadelphia: Lippincott Williams & Wilkins; 2009.

- Nemire RE, Kier KL, eds. *Pharmacy Clerkship Manual: A Survival Manual for Students.* New York: McGraw-Hill Medical Publishing; 2002.

Books on Communication Theory and Practice

- Patterson K, Grenny J, McMillan R, et al. *Crucial Conversations: Tools for Talking When the Stakes Are High.* New York: McGraw-Hill; 2002.

- James M, Jongeward D. *Born to Win: Transactional Analysis with Gestalt Experiments.* 25th anniversary ed. Cambridge, Mass: Perseus Books; 1996.

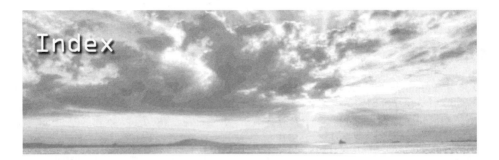

Index

Note: Page numbers followed by *f* and *t* indicate figures and tables, respectively.

K

L

M

T

tasks, student
    contribution to patients and site, 41
    creating and refining list of, 40–41
    linking value to objectives, 40–41
    timing of, 41
    "undesirable," avoiding pointing out, 41
teaching
    as art form, 61–64
    question-and-answer method of, problems in, 70–72
Teaching in Your Office: A Guide to Instructing Medical Students and Residents,
    2nd edition (Alguire et al., eds.), 134
technology, student use of
    as distraction, 93
    excessive, 111
telephone calls, excessive, 111
testing, formal, for students, 26–27
texting, excessive, 111
The Joint Commission (TJC), 16
timing
    of preceptor evaluation, 57
    of rotations, 9–10
    of student tasks, 41
TJC. *See* The Joint Commission

U

unfair advantage, students gaining, 122–123
unintended consequences, 70–72
unique aspects of practices, 63
unique knowledge, skills, and attitudes, 12–13
universities. *See* schools (colleges and universities)

V

verbal filter, lack of, 104–107
Veterans (generation), 73*t*
volunteering, 63–64

W

weekends, for making up missed time, 115
weighting, 20*f*, 25–26
"Who do I work for?" speech, 45
work, outside, as student distraction, 92
workload, number of students based on, 8–9
world view, of clinical training, 66–67, 66*f*
wrap-up feedback, from students, 53, 54

X

Y

APR 22 2003

One of the great advances of modern medicine is that expectant mothers can receive effective and safe pain relief during childbirth. **Childbirth and Pain Relief** *combines the best of several pain relief approaches and brings them together in an easy to understand book. The author, Dr. Sanjay Datta, is a world-recognized expert in this area; and has dedicated his entire professional career to improving both the safety and effectiveness of techniques to relieve pain in childbirth.*

—Robert Barbieri, M.D.
Kate Macy Ladd Professor of Obstetrics,
Gynecology and Reproductive Biology
Department of Obstetrics and Gynecology
Brigham and Women's Hospital

It is often difficult for women to make informed decisions concerning pain relief during childbirth given all the hearsay and misinformation out there. Dr. Datta, a world authority on obstetric anesthesia, has written a book, which goes a long way to present accurate information in a way that the lay reader can understand.

—Alan C. Santos, M.D., MPH,
Associate Director of Anesthesiology
St. Luke's-Roosevelt Hospital Center, New York

At last! A balanced approach to informing expectant parents about labor pain and their options for handling it. Well done, Dr. Datta.

—Gerard M. Bassell, M.D.
Editor-in-Chief, Obstetric Anesthesia Digest
Department of Anesthesiology
University of Kansas School of Medicine

The time has come in obstetrics. Parents should know the alternatives to the alleviation of pain during labor. They should be able to know truth from fiction. **Childbirth and Pain Relief** *provides a clear understanding to this complex problem.*

—Leonard E. Safon, M.D.
Clinical Associate Professor
Obstetrics and Gynecology
Harvard Medical School

Property of
Nashville Public Library
815 Church St., Nashville, Tn. 37219